Flat
Belly
Diet!®
For Men

Based on the *New York Times* best-selling diet

FROM THE EDITORS OF **Prevention**®

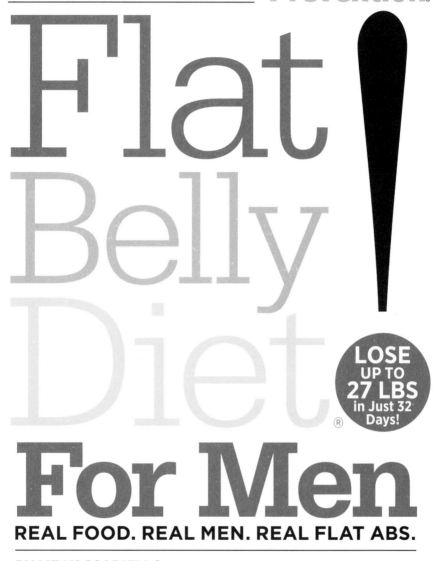

Flat Belly Diet! For Men

LOSE UP TO 27 LBS in Just 32 Days!

REAL FOOD. REAL MEN. REAL FLAT ABS.

BY LIZ VACCARIELLO, Editor-in-Chief, with D. Milton Stokes, MPH, RD

RODALE

Rodale books may be purchased for business or promotional
use or for special sales. For information, please write to:
Special Markets Department, Rodale Inc., 733 Third Avenue, New York, NY 10017

Prevention and Flat Belly Diet! are registered trademarks of Rodale Inc.

Printed in the United States of America

Rodale Inc. makes every effort to use acid-free ∞, recycled paper ♻.

Book design by Jill Armus and Maureen O'Brien
Exercise photos and Success Story photos by Steve Vaccariello
Food photos by Marcus Nilsson; Food styling by Anne Disrude;
Prop styling by Deborah Williams
Photo editing by Leah Vinluan

Library of Congress Cataloging-in-Publication Data
Flat belly diet! for men / Liz Vaccariello, editor-in-Chief, with D. Milton Stokes.
     p.   cm.
   Includes index.
   ISBN-13 978-1-60529-460-5 hardcover
   ISBN-10 1-60529-460-8 hardcover
   1. Reducing diets. 2. Abdomen. 3. Men—Health and hygiene. I. Vaccariello, Liz.
II. Stokes, D. Milton.
   RM222.2.F5324 2010
   613.2'5—dc22   2009044417

Distributed to the trade by Macmillan
2 4 6 8 10 9 7 5 3 1 hardcover

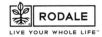

RODALE
LIVE YOUR WHOLE LIFE™

We inspire and enable people to improve their lives and the world around them
For more of our products visit **rodalestore.com** or call 800-848-4735

FOR THE FATHERS, SONS, BROTHERS,

AND HUSBANDS WHOSE HEALTH MATTERS

MORE THAN ANYTHING

—Liz and Milton

contents

acknowle

ACKNOWLEDGMENTS

dgments

WE DEDICATE THE Flat Belly Diet to the readers of *Prevention*—all 11 million of you—who have told us in no uncertain terms that belly fat is your biggest physical challenge.

Our gratitude to the Rodale family. For generations, through their magazines, books, and online properties, they have been committed to a special mission, that of giving people the tools and inspiration to live their whole lives. Our most heartfelt thanks to CEO Maria Rodale and former CEO Steve Murphy, whose leadership means Rodale is the kind of company where creativity is nurtured and the highest standards are set—and met—daily.

Like magazines, books are a collaborative effort, and this one is no exception. Very special thanks to Gregg Michaelson, Karen Rinaldi, Beth Lamb, Jenny Sucov, Bill Stump, and Marlea Clark, who were there at the beginning. To Robin Shallow, who never met an idea she didn't improve, and Bethridge Toovell and Lauren Paul, who are tireless in their enthusiasm, support, and belief in this plan. Thank you, Steve Madden, for, among other inspired ideas, Fire Water.

You would not be holding this book in your hands without editor Andrea au Levitt. All thanks to her dedicated team, including Marielle Messing, Carol Angstadt, Chris Krogermeier, Sara Cox,

JoAnn Brader, Hope Clarke, and Liz Krenos. We couldn't have crossed the finish line without Heather K. Jones's devotion to reenvisioning and revising this plan for men and David Bonom's dedication to creating delicious Flat Belly recipes. Many thanks also to Myatt Murphy for his cheerful professionalism and lightning-quick creation of a brand-new, guy-friendly, crunch-less exercise routine to flatten those abs. We'd also like to extend our gratitude to the original members of our initial test panel, which was conducted in the summer of 2009. Thank you, Anthony Henry, Neil Smith, Alan Musselman, John Rau, James Doherty, Mike Sauer, Phil DiScala, Nelson Duran, Will Pelkey, Joe Moscone, Joseph Tuckman, Robert Gray, and all their families for providing us with the essential insights that helped us develop this book beyond daily meal plans.

Big hugs to *Prevention*'s dazzling creative director, Jill Armus, and associate art director Maureen O'Brien, for their vision of *Flat Belly Diet! for Men*. And to *Prevention* fitness director Michele Stanten, who worked with Myatt to make Chapter 9 one of the most authoritative sources of information on banishing belly fat with exercise.

Thanks also to Lauren Parajon, who became best friends with our test panelists, and to Diana Kelly, Amanda Junker, and Greg Presto, who captured their enthusiasm and excitement on videotape. To Susan Graves, Courtenay Smith, and Polly Chevalier for their wise counsel and endless and sunny support. And to the smartest photo team in the business, including *Prevention*'s Helen Cannavale, Rebecca Simpson Steele, and Leah Vinluan. Our deep gratitude to original *Flat Belly Diet!* coauthor Cynthia Sass, MPH, RD, and former brand editor Leah McLaughlin, who were critical to developing the original plan upon which this is all based.

Finally, thank you to Steve Vaccariello—husband and photographer extraordinaire—who dropped 7 pounds in 4 days on the Four-Day Flat Abs Kickstart and convinced me that bellies of both sexes can and should be flattened! Speaking of families, kisses to Olivia and Sophia Vaccariello, and to Chef Kyle Shadix, MS, RD, Milton's restaurateur mom, Ann Stokes, and partner Bryan Giansanti—each a culinary expert—for helping brainstorm and test recipes. We love you all!

introd

uction

GET READY
FOR SIX-PACK ABS

IT'S NOT JUST women who struggle to keep their bellies flat. For better or worse, men are in the same boat when it comes to stubborn abdominal fat. Whether it's regularly pounding back beers with the guys, those killer cravings for fast food, or just plain old getting older, many men also start to see their waists expand.

I know firsthand that men—and their loved ones—are concerned about belly fat. As editor-in-chief of the leading US health magazine, *Prevention,* I constantly hear stories from women who have a love/hate relationship with their bellies. But after publishing *Flat Belly Diet!,* I quickly discovered that men are worried about this troublesome part of the body, too. Many of you told me that your growing gut was making you feel chunky and unattractive and that you want to feel ripped and fit.

Belly fat does not have to be your destiny. My book, *Flat Belly Diet!,* which became a *New York Times* bestseller as soon as it hit stores in October 2008, was the first diet to put into practice new research that monounsaturated fatty acids (aka MUFAs) target stubborn belly fat. We tested it on women, we watched while hundreds of thousands of readers got healthy—then we took the diet to Dr. David Katz at Yale to test out its health impact. As you'll learn in Chapter 1, the results wowed us all. And since powerful MUFAs can fight belly fat for women and men, I've adapted this effective eating plan for your needs and appetites, so you can lose weight, get healthy, and (you guessed it) flatten your belly, once and for all!

However, before I plunge into how this diet plan will work for you, it's important to look at why you've picked up this book in the first place. Since you bought this book, I'm guessing you want to eliminate that extra weight around your waist or perhaps even take it a step further and be the envy of your friends with a firm six-pack. Perhaps a woman in your life found success using the original *Flat Belly Diet!* book, and you want to see if it can work for you. Or, maybe, like my husband, Steve, you actually tried the original Flat Belly Diet and loved the results (Steve lost 8 pounds in 4 days!), but wished it addressed more of the weight loss challenges important to you: Can I lose weight without giving up alcohol? How do I stick to a diet when I have to entertain clients for work? Will I be able to build muscle at the same time I lose fat?

Whatever your motivation, your belly—and the rest of your body—will thank you for reading this book. It doesn't matter if your abs are rock hard or jiggly as Jell-O, they're the only set you have, and you need to work with them and respect them. Your belly is not only central to your confidence, but also to your health. Heart disease, diabetes, cancer—the biggest killers of men—are associated with excess fat around your middle. So saying adios to your gut will not only give you a lean body, it will also maximize your health.

After seeing the difference that *Flat Belly Diet!* made in the lives of millions of women, I embarked on a new quest to find the best way for men to eliminate belly fat. I teamed up with D. Milton Stokes, a prominent registered dietitian with over 20 years of experience in food and nutrition (10 of them specializing in weight management and sports nutrition), to create a plan that works for you. Milton took the science and successful eating plan from the original Flat Belly Diet and combined it with the latest research specific to weight loss for men plus his experience with his own clients to develop a diet that targets belly fat in men. He's spent countless hours helping men get into shape and stay lean. He knows what a growing gut can do to a man's self-confidence and his health, and he understands the weight loss challenges that men face every day. And as a former restaurateur, he knows that real men need real food, even (especially!) when they're on a diet. He has spent his career helping men combat this belly fat head-on.

Together we've developed a belly-shrinking, ab-flattening eating and exercise plan that works for men and is based on the latest and most credible science. It not only offers delicious, satisfying meals, but also provides new quick recipes to give you more options at work and on the go. If you want your abs to be not just flat but cut, there's even an all-new optional exercise program designed to give you that six-pack you've always wanted. The best part is that this plan will work for you whether this is your first time trying to lose weight or your 100th—whether you have never dieted or exercised before or have tried every weight loss program on the market. We tested it on real men with amazing results—our test panel of 12 men lost an average of more than 13 pounds and almost 9 inches over the course of just 32 days! The effects of the Flat Belly Diet for Men are long-lasting and work for all men, of all shapes and sizes, and all experience levels. And the tips, tricks, and strategies you'll learn in this book will teach you how to keep these healthy habits for life!

THE BASICS OF THE FLAT BELLY DIET FOR MEN

IT ALL STARTS with a few extra pounds around the waist. Next thing you know, you're trading up for a larger pair of pants, then suddenly your paunch is hanging over your new, bigger pants.

While this scenario might ring true for both men and women, the bad news for you guys is that it's more likely to happen to you. Yes, it's true. Men and women tend to put on excess weight differently, with guys being more prone to packing on the pounds around the waist.[1] Around 70 percent of American men are overweight or obese, and a lot of this excess flab is found on or around the belly.[2] Some scientists describe people with these love handles and belly fat as "apple shaped." Women, on the other hand, are often more "pear shaped," with a tendency to gain weight around their hips, thighs, and buttocks.

Having a spare tire can not only be bad for self-esteem—even if many men deny that they care—it also comes with serious health risks. Before we delve into how to flatten those abs, though, we need to take a closer look at this thing we're calling belly fat. All belly fat is not created equal; there are different kinds that can have different effects on your health.

Belly Fat: The Real Deal

THERE ARE ACTUALLY TWO TYPES of "belly fat" that can accumulate around your waist: subcutaneous and visceral. Subcutaneous fat, most simply and unscientifically put, is the fat you can see, the stuff you can actually grab. Subcutaneous means "beneath" (sub) "the skin" (cutaneous), so this easy-to-see fat is found all over the body—from your belly to the tips of your fingers.

Your body does need a moderate amount of subcutaneous fat to provide things such as energy and insulation during colder months. But having too much of it can be a visible sign that a person is overweight or obese, both of which are known to raise the risk for many diseases including heart disease, stroke, metabolic syndrome, certain types of cancer, type 2 diabetes, and sleep apnea.

The second type of fat is the more harmful kind. Visceral fat is found deep within the torso, and although some visceral fat is needed to protect the organs around the abdomen, too much can lead to big trouble. In fact, because of its proximity to your kidneys, heart, liver, and other organs, excess visceral fat can raise your risk of all sorts of diseases, from heart disease and diabetes to cancer and Alzheimer's. It's sometimes referred to as "hidden" belly fat because you can't see it from the outside, but I prefer the term "deadly" fat.

Here's the catch though: Cutting calories and upping your gym workouts doesn't necessarily guarantee that you'll lose a lot of visceral fat. And it's also possible to be "skinny fat"—to be relatively thin and still have too much visceral fat to be considered "healthy." It's enough to drive any guy nuts. The reality is that there's only one way to eat to minimize both visceral and subcutaneous fat simultaneously. To combat these fats you need to regularly eat, yes, fat . . . the right kind of fat, that is.

MUFAs: The Powerful Nutrient

CHANCES ARE YOU'VE HEARD of this fat-busting nutrient, or at the very least, you've eaten it. Monounsaturated fatty acids are found in oils, olives, nuts, and avocados, and we've known for decades that they have myriad health benefits. In fact, they are so popular they even have a nickname—MUFAs (pronounced MOO-fahs).

But it wasn't until the spring of 2007 that we realized just how amazing these fats are. That was when Spanish researchers published a study in the journal *Diabetes Care* that showed that eating a diet rich in MUFAs can actually help stop weight gain around the gut.[3]

The researchers looked at the effects of three diets—one high in saturated fat, another high in carbohydrates, and a third rich in MUFAs—on a group of patients with abdominal fat distribution, or, more simply, those with belly fat. All three diets had the same number of calories, but only the high-MUFA one was found to reduce the accumulation of belly fat, and, more specifically, visceral belly fat. This research showed that MUFAs are one of a kind, because no other nutrient has been found to aid ab flattening!

We used this science as the basis of the Flat Belly Diet, and that eating plan has helped—and continues to help—millions shed their belly fat. Now we've applied the same sound research to the Flat Belly Diet for Men. This is the only eating plan that helps you lose fat specifically in the belly, thanks to these powerful MUFAs.

According to a new Yale University Prevention Research Center Study, the Flat Belly Diet reduces dangerous visceral belly fat by an astonishing 33 percent. David L. Katz, MD, adjunct professor of public health and director of the

Yale Prevention Research Center at Yale University School of Medicine explains, "This diet study is exceptional because it shows the plan not only significantly reduces weight overall, but abdominal fat in particular, including dangerous visceral fat. We also saw impressive reductions in cholesterol, blood pressure, inflammation, and insulin resistance." The study participants, who followed the original Flat Belly Diet plan for 4 weeks, lost an average of 8.5 pounds, lowered their total cholesterol levels by more than 20 points, and reduced both systolic and diastolic blood pressure readings (by 8 points and 5 points, respectively). While the exact impact of these changes varies according to the individual, on average the Flat Belly Diet helped slash the risk of chronic diseases such as diabetes, heart disease, cancer, and arthritis by more than 50 percent!

You'll see that ab-flattening MUFAs are an essential part of the meals and snacks in this diet. Chapter 3 expands on the incredible power of MUFAs, but first let's take a closer look at how this unique plan works.

The Flat Belly Diet for Men Plan

THE FLAT BELLY DIET FOR MEN is made up of two parts—the Four-Day Flat Abs Kickstart, followed by the Four-Week MUFA Meal Plan. The whole thing takes just 32 days, which studies show is enough time to make any dietary change a part of your everyday lifestyle. And don't worry about the spare tire returning after the 32 days. Once you've mastered this program and watched your potbelly start to disappear, I will share the tools needed to keep your belly flat for life.

■ **THE FOUR-DAY FLAT ABS KICKSTART** isn't just about getting your body ready for flatter abs, it's also about getting your mind in the game. This part of the plan will get you into the habit of following the program and mentally prepare you for the next phase. The Four-Day Kickstart includes a prescribed list of foods and drinks that will help flush out fluid and relieve digestive issues like wind and constipation. You'll drink our signature Fire Water, which will help boost your metabolism, and eat healthy foods like fruits, vegetables, and whole grains.

Our initial test results were astonishing: One panelist—Neil—lost a whopping 7 pounds and a total of 8 inches from his body in just 4 days! He never dreamed it would be so easy. On average, the panelists lost 3.75 pounds and 2.91 inches during the Kickstart.

■ **THE FOUR-WEEK MUFA MEAL PLAN,** the real focus of this book, begins the morning after you finish the Flat Abs Kickstart. Every day for 28 days you'll enjoy three filling 400-calorie meals and two 400-calorie Power Snacks. Each meal and snack has just the right amount of MUFAs to help you flatten your abs and is chock-full of fiber and protein so you won't feel hungry, grouchy, or tired throughout the program. It really doesn't get any easier than this. There is no calorie counting, elimination of your favorite foods, or complicated rules. We picked 2,000 calories per day because that's how much an adult man of average height, frame, size, and activity level needs to get down to his ideal body weight while maintaining strong muscles and high energy levels. Upon completion of the 4-week segment, our panelists lost an average of 13.35 pounds and 8.86 inches total—2.81 inches from the abdominal area.

Customize Your Plan

FOR GUYS WHO DON'T have time to cook or just don't like cooking all that much, you'll find 90 MUFA-packed quick-fix meals, organized by breakfast, lunch, dinner, and snacks, in Chapter 7. Just choose three meals and two snacks a day and you're done. That's it! Chapter 8 is for days when you're feeling more ambitious with your meals. It includes more than 50 recipes for fast and delicious meals, each of which has the right number of calories and MUFAs per serving. There's even a grilling section in the chapter, which comes in handy for barbecue days, as well as easy-to-follow MUFA-related shopping and cooking tips. Don't like one of the meals? No problem. All of the meals are interchangeable so you never have to eat anything you don't like. Regardless of what meals you choose, you'll have flatter abs in a month, guaranteed.

To make life even easier, you'll see boxes called Fast Facts throughout the book. These boxes provide useful tidbits on fat, bulking up, weight loss, and general health, as well as quick tips and strategies. You'll also see some boxes labeled Message from Milton. Milton wrote these to share his advice and insight about how to achieve success on this incredible plan. To give you a little motivation if you're feeling discouraged, you'll even find amazing success stories from men who participated in our Flat Belly Diet for Men test panel and have a smaller paunch and tighter abs to prove it!

But what makes the Flat Belly Diet for Men truly special is that you don't need to exercise to reap the benefits. If you do exercise, you will certainly see results faster, and you will gain secondary benefits like improved cardiovascular health and stronger, more toned muscles. But you can still expect to shrink your belly—and lose both subcutaneous and visceral fat—by simply following the eating plan. I have always been a big believer in the phrase "small changes, big results." To me, it's more important that you do something to reduce your belly fat than it is to do everything, only to find that too many changes are difficult to maintain. If you do not already have a workout routine, incorporating a new way of eating into your lifestyle may be change enough for the first 32 days.

By the time you're done with this program, you'll not only feel fit and cut, but you'll have better health, more energy, and (of course!) those six-pack abs!

What about Exercise?

If you want to lose your belly fat *and* sculpt six-pack abs, exercise is going to get you there faster. I asked fitness expert Myatt Murphy, the author of *The Body You Want in the Time You Have*, *The Men's Health Gym Bible*, and *Men's Health Ultimate Dumbbell Guide*, to develop the exercise program in Chapter 9. This plan is doable, functional, and customizable to any fitness level, so even if it's been a while (or forever) since you've pumped iron or broken a sweat, Myatt's plan will get you in shape quickly and safely.

Flat Belly Diet for Men

→ The Four-Day Flat Abs Kickstart

Just 96 hours is all it takes to get you in the Flat Belly Diet game—and lose a few pounds! The Kickstart consists of:

■ **THREE SATISFYING 400-CALORIE MEALS** plus one easy-to-prepare 400-calorie snack.

■ **A DAILY DOSE OF MAKE-IN-ADVANCE FIRE WATER,** created by Milton to help guard against dehydration.

→ The Four-Week MUFA Meal Plan

Twenty-eight days of delicious MUFA-packed meals and recipes that you can mix and match. The plan consists of:

■ **THREE FILLING 400-CALORIE MEALS** and two 400-calorie Power Snacks. Choose from our quick-fix meal selections or recipes.

■ **A MUFA AT EVERY MEAL.** These super-healthy fats keep you feeling full and ensure every meal is exceptionally tasty.

→ An Optional Exercise Program

Build muscle, sculpt a six-pack, and maximize calorie burn with our fat-burning cardio plan plus the Maximum Metabolism Workout and Cut to the Core Routine.

READ A FLAT BELLY
SUCCESS
STORY

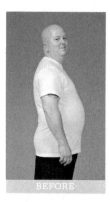

BEFORE

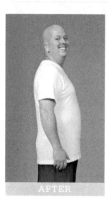

AFTER

Anthony Henry

AGE: 37

POUNDS LOST:

27.2

IN 32 DAYS

ALL-OVER
INCHES LOST:

15.75

3 FROM
THE WAIST

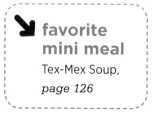

↘ favorite mini meal
Tex-Mex Soup,
page 126

"This plan has changed my life," says Anthony, a 37-year-old New York City firefighter at the firehouse closest to the World Trade Center. His life *and* his body. In just 35 days, Anthony lost an astounding 27.2 pounds and 15.75 inches overall—his family was awe-inspired by his physical transformation. And considering Anthony's lifelong battle with his weight, so was he.

"I didn't start off as the heavy kid," he explains. "I was rail thin up until seventh grade. But by age 15, I stopped growing *up* and started growing *out*." By age 17, Anthony was 15 pounds overweight; by age 30, 40 pounds overweight. He had tried every fad diet on the market—all punctuated events with clear starting and stopping points. He would drop a few pounds when he needed to (to pass the firefighter test, for instance), but, inevitably, gain them all back, over and over again.

"I was not chubby, husky, or a few pounds overweight—I was really heavy," says Anthony. "And I would get ridiculed at work because of it. Everywhere you turn in my firehouse there is some sort of picture mocking my appearance due to my weight. It was embarrassing, but instead of spurring me on to make a change, it drove me to eat more and do less. I'd even ridicule myself to beat them to the punch and take the sting out of it. As the weight came off and the guys saw me lose weight, the jokes turned to praise. Now they ask me how to make their meals healthier."

His 3-year-old daughter, Ella Kate, helped motivate him to make a change. "My desire to lose weight had a lot to do with her. I told myself that I had to get in shape for my new child. I have gone to fires where I've had to climb 14 stories with over 100 pounds of gear and *then* go to work. I didn't want to die of a heart attack climbing up the stairs to a fire."

Anthony's success while on the Flat Belly Diet for Men was tied to planning ahead. Plain and simple. "If you don't give it some thought ahead of time, how can you make good choices? Nutrition doesn't just magically happen." He made shopping lists, mapped out his meals, and made a game plan for his daily food choices.

Anthony also adopted a healthier mindset. "I stopped looking at the final day of this plan as the work being complete or the process being over," explains Anthony. "I realize this is something I have to do every day. I can eat whatever I want, but I have to do it in moderation. And I also have to continue with my fitness regimen. I don't see this as a "diet," like the nasty four-letter word. I see it as a lifestyle change that I'm finally ready to accept." Anthony feels prepared now for new challenges, especially those involving physical activity. His wife sees it, too. "He's definitely more confident now that he's changed his eating and lost weight."

Anthony used this plan to turn his life around. Next up for Anthony: training for and running a half marathon to benefit the Crohn's and Colitis Foundation of America.

THE 411 ON BELLY FAT

BODY FAT MAY get a bad rep, but you actually need some to survive. Without fat, your body would essentially fall apart. Why? This fat insulates your body from the cold and the heat, while protecting your internal organs from outside damage. It allows your organs to produce the hormones that make you distinctly male. It's necessary as backup energy when your blood sugar runs out. It helps your cells hold together and absorb nutrients from the food you eat.

And that's just the beginning of the long list of useful things done by body fat. Basically, you wouldn't be the man you are today if it weren't for fat, since it plays a role in nearly every single biological function in your body. It's impossible to live without it. But there can be too much of a "good" thing, and a fine line exists between just the right amount of body fat and having too much.

Gauging Your Gut

THE DANGERS OF EXCESS BODY FAT, whether it's in your gut or hefty arms or legs, have been recognized for some time now. Obesity—which, technically speaking, means to be "overfat"—is considered to be as deadly as smoking, according to some analyses. Weighing yourself will give you some sense of how heavy you are, but it doesn't actually show how fat you are. The body mass index (BMI), a common measurement based on weight and height, is more useful for working this out. Here's how to calculate it.

- Multiply your weight in pounds by 703.
- Divide that number by your height in inches.
- Divide that number by your height in inches again.

A man who weighs 170 pounds and is 72 inches tall (6 feet), for instance, has a BMI of 23.1. A man who weighs 300 pounds and is 72 inches tall has a BMI

HEIGHT	WEIGHT (LB)													
5'0"	97	102	107	112	118	123	128	133	138	143	148	153	158	163
5'1"	100	106	111	116	122	127	132	137	143	148	153	158	164	169
5'2"	104	109	115	120	126	131	136	142	147	153	158	164	169	175
5'3"	107	113	118	124	130	135	141	146	152	158	163	169	175	180
5'4"	110	116	122	128	134	140	145	151	157	163	169	174	180	186
5'5"	114	120	126	132	138	144	150	156	162	168	174	180	186	192
5'6"	118	124	130	136	142	148	155	161	167	173	179	186	192	198
5'7"	121	127	134	140	146	153	159	166	172	178	185	191	198	204
5'8"	125	131	138	144	151	158	164	171	177	184	190	197	203	210
5'9"	128	135	142	149	155	162	169	176	182	189	196	203	209	216
5'10"	132	139	146	153	160	167	174	181	188	195	202	209	216	222
5'11"	136	143	150	157	165	172	179	186	193	200	208	215	222	229
6'0"	140	147	154	162	169	177	184	191	199	206	213	221	228	235
6'1"	144	151	159	166	174	182	189	197	204	212	219	227	235	242
6'2"	148	155	163	171	179	186	194	202	210	218	225	233	241	249
BMI	19	20	21	22	23	24	25	26	27	28	29	30	31	32

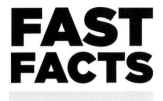

FAST FACTS

We're all born with the same number of fat cells (about 40 billion, give or take). As we grow up, the number of fat cells we have increases until after our pubescent and adolescent years, when they are pretty much set. In the past, it was assumed that the only difference between overweight people and thin ones was that overweight or obese people had all their fat cells filled to maximum capacity. It's now known that we can—and do, in fact—"grow" more fat cells in adulthood. This is because when fat cells expand to their maximum size, they divide and increase the number of fat cells. Some obese people have more fat cells than non-obese people. But in the end, both the number and the size of the fat cells determine the amount of fat someone has.

of 40.7. You can also visit prevention.com and search for "BMI calculator" for an instant calculation or consult the chart on the opposite page.

If your BMI is 25 or higher, you're considered to be overweight, and if it's 30 or above, you're classified as obese. Your health is at greatest risk if your BMI is 40 or more, since this is considered morbidly obese. Too low a BMI isn't good either. A BMI below 18.5 is considered underweight, indicating that you have too low a percentage of body fat to ensure healthy functioning. What you want is a number between 18.5 and 24.9 (in black on the chart).

You may have heard that doesn't account for muscle mass. Many professional athletes, for instance, have a higher percentage of muscle compared to body fat and therefore have a relatively high BMI. While the BMI does have limitations and should not be used by men who are competitive athletes, bodybuilders, or chronically ill patients, for most of you reading this book, it is an effective tool to gauge health risk related to weight.

A bigger problem with BMI, however, is that it doesn't reveal how much fat you're carrying around the belly. This is really important information, especially for guys, who tend to be more gut-prone than women. Recent studies show that while general obesity is unhealthy, carrying excess body fat specifically around the waist is really, *really* unhealthy. These studies show that men with waistlines measuring 40 inches or more are at greater risk for heart disease and diabetes than those with smaller guts.[1] (For women, a waistline of 35 inches or more indicates the same health risks.) Heart disease is the number one killer of American men (as well as the biggest killer of women), and diabetes has reached alarming rates among men.[2] Twelve million (or 11.2 percent) of adult men in the United States have diabetes, although nearly one-third of them don't know it.[3] The connection between the measurement of your waist and your risk of dying from one of these diseases isn't a coincidence.

What's to Blame?

IF YOU DO DISCOVER that you're overweight or obese, it's easy to find things to fault. There's the fried chicken, perhaps, or that six-pack of beer you consume regularly. Not to mention the nachos, chicken wings, and a daily diet of processed or fast food. The truth is, eating or drinking too much of anything that's a source of extra calories (including, but not limited to, beer) will make you gain weight and lead to the dreaded "beer" (aka fat) belly.

Genetics can also play a role in the size of your gut. Your genes can impact

The Blood Lipids

There are several types of cholesterol, but in most cases, the American Heart Association concentrates on two—namely, HDL and LDL.

LDL is known as the "bad" cholesterol because it builds up on artery walls and can lead to increased risk for cardiovascular disease and stroke. The American Heart Association considers a level of 130 mg/dL (milligrams per deciliter of blood) or less optimal for most people.

HDL is the healthy cholesterol. It transports LDL cholesterol out of the bloodstream and deposits it in the liver, where it can be processed and excreted. High amounts of HDL (60 mg/dL or higher) give some protection from heart disease.

The ratio of HDL to total cholesterol is a

your chances of being overweight or obese, as well as where this extra fat ends up on your body.[4] The reality for most men, though, is that their big belly has more to do with lifestyle than heredity. While muscle mass naturally decreases with age, as men get older they also tend to cut back on physical activity. They're likely to eat a little more and work out a lot less. Considering that muscle loss slows the rate at which your body burns calories, these unhealthy habits are a surefire way to pack on the pounds. And if you're not limiting your caloric intake or upping your workouts as you age, chances are you'll gain weight.

To make matters worse, as we've learned, men are naturally disadvantaged when it comes to their guts. Men and women typically gain excess weight differently, with guys being more prone to packing on the pounds around the waist— called apple shaped. Female body fat, on the other hand, often concentrates around the hips, thighs, and buttocks, making them pear shaped. Men actually have twice as much fat around the abdominal cavity (or less scientifically put, around the stomach) as women.[5] Hormones may be partly to blame for this disparity. Lower-body fat cells are more responsive to the hormone estrogen, found in higher levels in women, whereas abdominal fat is more responsive to the stress hormone adrenaline.[6] Another reason for this difference may be related to a gene that codes for lipoprotein lipase (LPL), an enzyme made by fat cells to help store

very good way of measuring cardiovascular risk. Most physicians consider a ratio of 4 or under excellent. A person with total cholesterol of 200 mg/dL and an HDL of 50 mg/dL (total/HDL ratio = 4) has a lower risk of heart disease and stroke than someone with a total of 180 mg/dL and an HDL of 30 mg/dL (total/HDL ratio = 6).

Triglycerides (another type of fat found in the blood) should also be considered. Several studies indicate that men (and women) who have high triglyceride levels, along with high LDL cholesterol, may increase their chances of having heart disease more than having only high LDL cholesterol levels.[7] The National Cholesterol Education Program sets guidelines for safe triglycerides that are less than 150 milligrams per deciliter (mg/dL).

calories as fat. In women, fat cells in the hips, thighs, and breasts secrete LPL, while in men it's produced by fat cells in the belly area.[8]

Perils of Visceral Fat

THOUGH THERE ARE DIFFERENT types of fat in the belly, there's one in particular that you should be worried about: visceral fat.

Some people call this the hidden fat because it's sequestered under a layer of muscle and doesn't show up on your gut (or anywhere else for that matter). This makes things tricky because you can be gutless and still have too much visceral fat. It's hard to imagine that a guy may be lean and fat at the same time, but Jimmy Bell, PhD, a professor of molecular imaging at Imperial College, London, has shown that it is possible. Dr. Bell and his team have been using magnetic resonance imaging (MRI) machines to scan nearly 800 people in an effort to produce what they call "fat maps." His findings are surprising: About 65 percent of the lean men and 45 percent of the thin women he tested carried excess visceral fat.[9]

Knowing how much visceral fat you have is vital because this fat can be deadly and can subtract years from your life. Carrying excess visceral fat is one of a complex group of symptoms collectively called metabolic syndrome, or syn-

How Fat Cells Work

A fat cell is like a small, expandable capsule—so small in fact that it can only hold a microscopic drop of fat. But fat cells don't like to live alone; they cluster together like mobs to become fatty tissue. They generally just hang out until they're called into action by precise biochemical signals, usually hormones and enzymes. These hormones and enzymes signal fat into the bloodstream to be used for different purposes.

When you overeat, those extra calories will travel right back into those deflated fat cells and fill them back up. No matter how much weight you lose or how many hours you spend lifting weights, your fat cells will never disappear. A deflated balloon is still a balloon.

drome X. The other symptoms are abnormal cholesterol, high blood pressure, and elevated insulin levels. Having just one of these conditions contributes to your risk of serious disease, and your risk grows exponentially as the number of symptoms increase.

Visceral fat has been linked to a long list of adverse health conditions, the most serious of which are

- High blood pressure, stroke, and heart disease
- Diabetes
- Dementia

One of the main reasons visceral fat is so deadly is its role in inflammation, a natural immune response that has recently been linked to almost every chronic disease out there. Visceral fat secretes precursors to an inflammatory chemical, which helps fuel the systemic process that exacerbates early symptoms of a disease.

Another reason why too much of this fat is so damaging may be related to its location near the portal vein, which carries blood from the intestinal area to the liver. When visceral fat releases substances, such as free fatty acids, they can enter the portal vein, make their way to the liver, and influence what blood lipids are produced.[10] This may be why visceral fat is linked to a negative impact on blood lipids. One study in the *New England Journal of Medicine* found that people with large bellies produce lower levels of HDL cholesterol, the "healthy" kind, than people with large hips and small waists.[11] Men typically have lower HDL levels, which is linked to more heart attacks, than women. Besides producing lower HDL levels, having a lot of visceral fat has been associated with higher total and higher LDL cholesterol levels.[12]

This bad-for-you fat also contributes to insulin resistance, an early precursor to diabetes. Insulin resistance is a condition in which cells do not respond normally to the hormone insulin, so the pancreas is forced to increase production to clear the bloodstream of the sugar glucose. Over time, insulin resistance can lead to full-blown diabetes, which can severely compromise the entire circulatory system and cause long-term issues with vision, memory, and wound healing, among other things.

Unfortunately, it doesn't stop there. Visceral fat not only impacts the body, it can apparently affect the mind, too. A study by Kaiser Permanente compared people with different levels of abdominal fat. The results showed that those who had the most abdominal fat were 145 percent more likely to develop dementia than people with the least amount of abdominal fat.[13] The researchers blamed this on inflammation.

A Fundamental Figure

THE NATIONAL INSTITUTES OF HEALTH (NIH) has stated that a waist measurement of more than 40 inches for men (and 35 inches for women) is an unhealthy sign of excess visceral fat—no matter what your weight on the scale.[14]

One simple way to assess the amount of fat around your gut is called the *waist-to-hip ratio.* Though this measurement doesn't reveal if you are overweight, it is slightly more targeted to belly fat—and this is a vital thing to know. Scientists who analyzed data from 27,000 people in 52 countries found that heart attack sufferers had BMIs similar to, but waist-to-hip ratios higher

The Benefits of Fat

From 2 to 5 percent of a man's body weight comes from essential fat. Fat is essential in humans for:

- Energy
- Maintaining proper hormone levels
- Regulating body temperature
- Protecting vital organs
- Fertility
- Bone growth

Body fat only becomes a problem when there's too much of it. At that point, it puts a strain on your heart and other organs and starts to interfere with your body confidence.

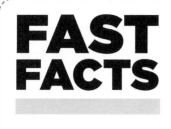
than, those who'd never had a heart attack. So which number would you rather track?

The best part about the waist-to-hip ratio is that it's easy to calculate. All you need is a measuring tape to compare the narrowest part of your waist to the broadest section of your hips. Your waist measurement should be taken in the spot between the ribcage and the hipbone, as viewed from the front. Be sure your abdomen is bare and that the tape is snug (but doesn't compress your skin) and parallel to the floor. Your hip measurement is most accurate if you turn sideways to the mirror and incorporate your rear end in the measurement. Now divide your waist measurement by your hip measurement.

A man with a 36-inch waist and 37-inch hips, for example, would have a waist/hip ratio of 0.97. According to the Centers for Disease Control and Prevention, a healthy waist-to-hip ratio for men should not exceed 0.90.[16] This is the essential number you must remember.

Other Ways to Measure Visceral Fat

The fact that people can have high amounts of visceral fat despite being at a normal weight (essentially those who are lean on the outside but have excess fat on the inside) is a relatively new idea. As we understand more about the dangers of visceral fat, researchers are developing increasingly accurate—and expensive—ways to measure it. Some of these methods include the following:

TESTING FOR RBP4 One of the latest tests out there, it detects levels of a protein called *retinol binding protein 4* (RBP4). This protein is produced in higher quantities in visceral fat compared with subcutaneous fat. In overweight people, blood levels of RBP4 are double or triple the amounts found in normal-weight people.

BIOELECTRICAL IMPEDANCE ANALYSIS Bioelectrical impedance analysis (BIA) is portable, easy to use, and low-cost compared with other procedures. A BIA involves circulating a very faint electrical current through the body. A device then calculates the resistance the current encounters as it travels through the body, computing body fat percentage based on height, weight, and speed of the current. A faster current translates to a lower body fat percentage because electricity travels faster through muscle (a greater percentage of water is found in muscle) than through fat. In addition to taking waist and hip measurements, this is the method we used to measure visceral fat in our test panelists.

SONOGRAM/ULTRASOUND Ultrasound machines send out high-frequency sound waves that reflect off body structures of different densities to create a picture called a *sonogram*. There is no radiation exposure with this test. A clear, water-based conducting gel is applied to the skin over the area being examined to improve the transmission of the sound waves. The ultrasound transducer (a hand-held probe) is then moved over the abdomen to produce an image of what's inside.

DEXA Dual-energy X-ray absorptiometry (DEXA) uses less radiation than a CT scan (see oposite page) to assess visceral fat and is less expensive. It's typically used to assess bone mineral density but can also be a valuable tool in assessing body composition.

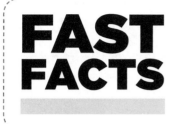

MRI Magnetic resonance imaging (MRI) uses powerful magnets and radio waves to create pictures without the use of radiation. Images generated by MRI are generally superior to—but also usually more expensive than—computed tomography (see below) because they are more finely detailed.

CT SCAN A computed tomography (CT or CAT) scanner uses radiation to create cross-sectional pictures of the body. The image results in a cross section of your belly that shows very clearly how much fat surrounds your organs. The latest scanners can image a whole body in less than 30 seconds.

Getting Past Your Gut

REMEMBER, YOU CAN MOST easily determine if your belly is potentially endangering your health with just an inexpensive tape measure. But even if your belly measurement doesn't indicate that your health is at risk, I'm guessing you still want to transform your flabby middles into rock-hard abs. And there's another reason—besides protecting your health and flattening your gut—for trying this plan: the delicious food! In the next chapter, you'll learn more about MUFAs, the powerful nutrient that makes the Flat Belly Diet for Men effective, easy, and delicious.

READ A FLAT BELLY
SUCCESS
STORY

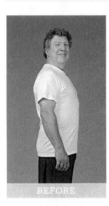

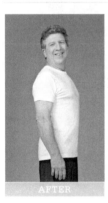

Neil Smith

AGE: 60

POUNDS LOST:

22.6

IN 32 DAYS

ALL-OVER
INCHES LOST:

13.88

3.5 FROM
THE WAIST

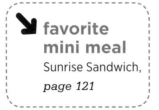

↘ **favorite mini meal**
Sunrise Sandwich,
page 121

"It's been 15 years, or more, since I was under 200 pounds! I fit the classic one-or-two-pounds-a-year-since-college mold," says 60-year-old Neil, a semiretired dentist who is busy building a new home in Washington state. His daughter, Ella, a nutrition student at Hunter College in New York City, learned about the Flat Belly Diet for Men test panel through her school and encouraged her dad to partici-pate. Neil went all out. Now, almost 23 pounds lighter and 14 inches slimmer than when he began the plan, Neil is the second most successful panelist.

"The Four-Day Flat Abs Kick-start was especially easy to follow. I enjoy precision, so weighing and measuring what I ate, although new, came easy." During the Kickstart, Neil lost a whopping 7.1 pounds and 8.25 inches overall. "My wife appreciated the immedi-ate results of the Kickstart and my obvious improving health, which happened right away in the Kickstart." And then he just kept on losing . . . and losing . . . until he was down nearly 23 pounds from his starting weight.

Neil's wife, Elaine, had faith in her husband. "I knew he could do it. He was motivated by the scientific aspect of the plan." Elaine also explained that Neil had an easy go of it because they had most of the Flat Belly–approved foods in the house already. The difference in his cooking style? Pausing for just a second to measure out ingredients rather than just eyeballing the amounts. "This plan empowered me," he said. "It showed me that cooking healthfully, which includes actually measuring, is easy and fast." Elaine chimed in, saying, "Neil became an expert at determining how much a proper serving contained. He could grab the exact amount of almonds for his snack. Beforehand, I think he was out of touch with what a healthy portion was supposed to be."

Another Flat Belly trick for Neil is planning ahead. With his wife's encouragement and help, Neil set aside time routinely to plan his meals and snacks. "When I was going to be away from home working on the new house or out running errands, I would pack a snack. This way I didn't get too hungry and stop to eat the first thing I saw."

Like other panelists, Neil's had to go clothes shopping for a smaller size. He says, "I actually had to punch new holes in my belts or my old pants would slide right off!"

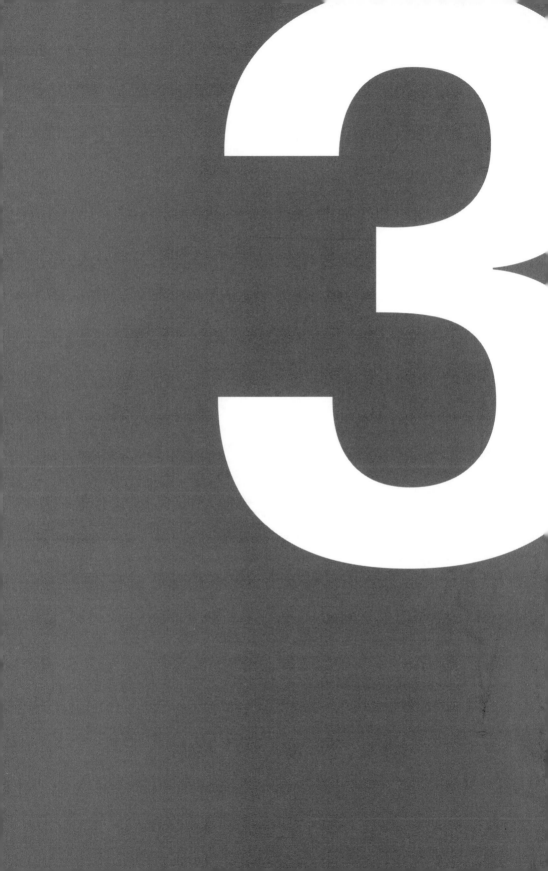

THE POWER OF MUFAs

THERE ARE NO two ways about it—belly fat is dangerous. But here's the good news: You don't have to live with it. You don't need to spend another day feeling uncomfortable about your gut hanging over your pants or worrying about your rising health risks. Why? There's a simple solution to your spare tire: MUFAs. There are five categories of MUFAs.

> **1. OILS**
> **2. OLIVES**
> **3. NUTS AND SEEDS**
> **4. AVOCADOS**
> **5. DARK CHOCOLATE**

These super foods hold the power to transform your body and your life. How, you may wonder? It's all in the name. "MUFA" stands for monounsaturated fatty acid. It's a mouthful, I know, but the tongue twister describes exactly why these plant-based fats are so healthy.

Sticks and Strings

FATTY ACIDS ARE BASICALLY the building blocks of all dietary fats. Like all organic elements, they're made up of carbon, oxygen, and hydrogen atoms lined up in a particular order to form a chain. The term *saturated* is used when every carbon atom in the chain is bound to a hydrogen atom. This makes them solid or waxy at room temperature and sticky and inflexible in your body. Unsaturated fats aren't so tightly constructed, allowing them to be more flexible. This flexibility is the basis for why unsaturated fats are considered "good" and saturated fats are "bad."

Here's an easy way to keep it straight: Think of saturated fats as sticks and unsaturated fats as strings. As saturated fats travel through your arteries, they

Good Fat versus Bad Fat

Dietary fat is an important energy source. Used in the production of cell membranes and certain hormones, it's critical to the regulation of blood pressure, heart rate, blood vessel constriction, blood clotting, and the nervous system. Dietary fat aids the body in absorbing vitamins such as A, D, E, and K. But not all fats are created equal. Eating large amounts of the wrong fat is very hazardous to your health. But telling good fats from bad ones isn't so easy, unless you know what to look for. Here's a quick guide to the fats you hear about most often.

THE HEALTHY

MONOUNSATURATED FAT (MUFA) remains liquid at room temperature but may start to solidify in the refrigerator.
POLYUNSATURATED FAT remains in liquid form both at room temperature and in the refrigerator. Foods high in polyunsaturated fats include vegetable oils, such as safflower, corn (maize), sunflower, and soya oils.
OMEGA-3 FATTY ACIDS are an exceptionally healthy type of polyunsaturated fat found mostly in fat-rich seafoods such as salmon, mackerel, and herring. If

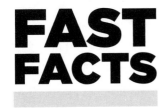
bump and grind their way through and often get stuck along the way. A study published in the *Journal of the American College of Cardiology* found that eating a meal high in saturated fat reduced the ability of blood vessels to expand and impaired blood flow.[1] This effect happened just 3 hours after eating. That's not the only downside. Numerous studies have linked a long-term high intake

you'd rather do your tax return than eat two fish meals a week (the recommended intake of healthy seafood), walnuts, flaxseeds (linseeds), flaxseed (linseed) oil, and, to a lesser degree, rapeseed (canola) oil also contain omega-3 fatty acids.

THE UNHEALTHY

SATURATED FATS become solid or semisolid at room temperature. The marbling in red meat is one example, as is a pat of butter. Saturated fat is found mostly in animal foods, but three vegetable sources are also high in saturated fat: coconut oil, palm (or palm kernel) oil, and cocoa butter. Keep in mind that it's almost impossible to get your saturated fat intake down to zero. Even olive oil contains 2 grams of saturated fat per tablespoon.

TRANS FATS raise LDL cholesterol and lower HDL cholesterol, increasing the risk of heart disease. They're quite possibly the most hated fats in all of fat-dom. Created when manufacturers hydrogenate liquid oils to increase their shelf life, they're found mostly in packaged products and nearly every food that contains shortening. Look out for the words "hydrogenated" or "partially hydrogenated" on ingredients lists to locate—and avoid—deadly trans fats.

of saturated fat to an increased risk of atherosclerosis (hardening of the arteries), heart disease, stroke, and other chronic diseases.

Since MUFAs are unsaturated (the more flexible kind), they can easily glide through your bloodstream without gumming up the works. This flexibility is just one reason why MUFAs are so healthful; a growing body of research indicates they may actually help unclog and protect arteries from buildup.

The MUFA Story

To REALLY UNDERSTAND WHY "a MUFA at every meal" is an integral part of the Flat Belly Diet for Men, let's briefly recap the history of these powerful fats and see how they rose to nutritional stardom. Understanding this history will provide perspective on just how far we've come, fats-wise.

At one time, not that long ago, all fats were sort of lumped together in the "bad" or "fattening" category. In the 1950s, recommendations were introduced from health professionals and the government based on the relationship between fats and heart disease.[2] Ever since then, these guidelines have empha-

Say No to Trans Fat

These man-made fats are created from vegetable oils in a process called *partial hydrogenation,* which adds hydrogen to liquid unsaturated oils. This changes their structure into a form that helps hold ingredients together in foods like pie crusts, biscuits, or crackers. Because trans fats spoil more slowly, they extend a product's shelf life. Research shows that not only are trans fats bad for your heart because they clog arteries and raise "bad" LDL cholesterol, but they also increase the accumulation of belly fat, according to US research. To avoid trans fats, look at the Nutrition Facts panel on labels, and check the ingredients lists. Labels are allowed to list trans fat as zero grams if they contain less than half a gram per serving. If the words *partially hydrogenated* appear, limit or avoid the food—even if it says "zero grams of trans fat."

sized lowering saturated fat specifically, while the overall message has been to reduce total fat intake. One of the main tenets of the 1980 Dietary Guidelines was: "Avoid too much fat, saturated fat, and cholesterol."[3] These government guidelines are revised every 5 years, but that wording stayed put for the next three versions. A full 15 years later, the 1995 report still stated, "Fat, whether from plant or animal sources, contains more than twice the number of calories of an equal amount of carbohydrate or protein. Choose a diet that provides no more than 30 percent of total calories from fat."[4]

This emphasis on total fat and the "no more than 30 percent" wording led many men and women to believe that "the less the better." The result? Scores of fat-phobic consumers began avoiding not only butter and well-marbled meats, but also vegetable oils, nuts, and peanut butter.

Let's jump ahead to the year 2000. The Dietary Guidelines of that year were slightly less restrictive. They stated, "Choose a diet that is low in saturated fat and cholesterol and moderate in total fat" and mentioned the healthfulness of plant-based fats, including oils and nuts.[5] But the message "Aim for a total fat intake of no more than 30 percent of calories" still remained. It wasn't until a few years ago, in the 2005 Dietary Guidelines, that a minimum fat recommendation finally appeared.[6] The wording about fat in this version of the guidelines states, "Keep total fat intake between 20 to 35 percent of calories, with most fats coming from sources of polyunsaturated and monounsaturated fatty acids."

"Fat Free" Fuels Obesity

Studies from the 1950s to 1970s had indicated that a high total fat intake was associated with a greater risk of cardiovascular disease (CVD). According to the American Heart Association, CVD has been the number one killer in the United States every year for more than a century, except during the 1918 flu pandemic.[7] And population data showed that Americans were consuming over a third of their total calories from fat. The 1971 National Health and Nutrition

Examination Survey (NHANES) found that American men consumed 36.1 percent of total calories from fat, while women ate 36.9 percent.[8]

The message to reduce fat intake worked—well, kind of. By 2000, that percentage dropped to 32.8 percent for both men and women. Trouble is, total fat consumption in grams actually increased! The percentage shrank because total calorie intake rose—from roughly 2,450 calories to 2,618 for men and from about 1,542 calories to 1,877 for women. Most of these extra calories came from carbohydrates, causing the percentage of fat in the diet to shrink. According to the data, carbohydrate intake jumped by a whopping 68 grams per day among men and 62 grams among women, while total fat decreased among men by 5.3 grams and increased among women by 6.5 grams.

Maybe you recall the hype from around this time, when fat-free, high-carb foods were flying off the shelves. It was nearly impossible to avoid these products at the grocery store, and both men and women couldn't get enough of them. With all this emphasis on fat, most people saw a green light to eat large quantities of fat-free foods (like entire boxes of cookies and gigantic plates of pasta). And guess what? Obesity rates began to skyrocket, rising from 14.5 percent in 1971 to 30.9 percent in 2000.

"Good" Fats Finally Surface

Clearly, the "eat less fat" message wasn't working. So in the 1990s, scientists started to pay attention to a theory that eating moderate amounts of some types of fats could be beneficial.

This idea was first proposed in a report known as the Seven Countries Study, by University of Minnesota scientist Ancel Keys, PhD.[9] Between 1958 and 1970, Keys and colleagues followed populations of men ages 40 to 59 in 18 areas of seven countries (United States, Japan, Italy, Greece, the Netherlands, Finland, and Yugoslavia). The study looked at the men's diets, disease risk factors (such as blood cholesterol levels and blood pressure), and disease rates. It was the first

FAST FACTS

A calorie is a unit of energy needed to increase the temperature of 1 gram of water by 1°C. In everyday terms, it's energy that can have one of four origins and one of three destinations. There are four sources of calories: carbohydrates, protein, fat, and alcohol. The first three types are essential to the body, but alcohol is not. When one of these types becomes available to the body, the cells will do one of three things with this energy. Basically, there is a priority system.

Fuel is the number one priority of every cell in the body. Just like cars need gasoline, cells need fuel to perform their jobs (breathing, circulation, movement, etc.). Carbohydrate calories are the cells' preferred source of energy. The next priority is repair, healing, and maintenance. Your body takes the energy from proteins and fats and uses it to patch up cells that are damaged or to create new cells. Your muscles, bones, skin, and immune system rely on protein and fat energy for this work. Finally, if all the cells are properly fueled and repaired or replaced, your body takes the leftover or unneeded energy and stores it in your fat cells.

When your body is in "energy balance," the number of calories that showed up for work (the amount eaten) matched your needs perfectly. If you're in a positive energy balance, too many showed up, and you ended up storing some (i.e., weight gain). A negative energy balance means not enough calories are available. This can result in fatigue, feeling run-down, and getting sick or injured. The Flat Belly Diet for Men is designed to keep you in balance—it provides enough energy in the form of carbohydrates, proteins, and fats, but not too much.

study to look at the links between diets and disease outcomes in different populations. This study was important because it demonstrated the degree to which the composition of a diet could predict rates of coronary heart disease. The major conclusion—finally!—was that a high fat intake was not associated with higher rates of heart disease.

The area that stuck out in Keys's studies was Crete, the largest of the Greek islands. Cretan men had the lowest rates of heart disease of all the populations observed in the Seven Countries Study, as well as the longest average life span, despite consuming 37 percent of their calories from fat. (Finland and the United States had the highest number of deaths from heart disease.)

Throughout the study, Keys observed that the Cretans' diets were consistent. They consumed the same types of traditional Greek meals they had enjoyed for centuries, including lots of fruits, vegetables (especially greens), nuts, beans, fish, moderate amounts of wine and cheese, small quantities of grass-fed meat, milk, eggs, some whole grains, and plenty of MUFA-rich olive oil and olives. Cretan people consume on average 25 liters (100 cups) of olive oil per person each year.

An Ode to Olive Oil

The fascinating findings in Crete put olive oil at center stage, fueling the idea that some fats are healthful. Dozens of Mediterranean diet studies focusing on olive oil followed, with amazing conclusions. A Greek study found that the exclusive use of olive oil was associated with a 47 percent lower likelihood of having CVD, even after adjustments were made to account for BMI, smoking, physical activity level, educational status, a family history of heart disease, high blood pressure, high cholesterol, and diabetes.[10] Another study published in the *American Journal of Clinical Nutrition* in the late 1990s looked at the effects of long-term olive oil intake and blood triglyceride levels on a group of healthy men.[11] The olive oil group had significantly reduced levels of LDL cholesterol.

As research on this topic grew, we learned more and more about the potential benefits of olive oil. Numerous controlled studies have found that it can lower circulating LDL levels and prevent cholesterol from hardening. That's critical, because hardening kicks off the domino effect that results in artery damage and disease. But as more and more studies were conducted, it became clear that while olive oil is extremely healthful, a great deal of its protective power lies in its MUFAs, which are also found in other plant fats such as nuts and avocado.

What Can MUFAs Do for You?

Eventually, research shifted from olive oil to MUFAs, and it was discovered that MUFA protection extends far beyond cholesterol and heart disease. MUFAs have now been linked to reduced rates of type 2 diabetes, metabolic syndrome, prostate cancer, and inflammation, plus healthier blood pressure, brain function, lung function, body weight, and—you guessed it—belly fat. In fact, when I saw the stacks and stacks of published studies on MUFAs, I was stunned. So in the interest of not overwhelming you (and saving you a lot of time!), I've included a few of the most compelling studies. I think this summary will help you see why we're so excited about MUFAs.

MUFAs Provide Heart Protection

Cardiovascular diseases (which include coronary heart disease, stroke, high blood pressure, and rheumatic heart disease) are the number one cause of death for men in the United States. About one in three adult men has some form of heart disease. The good news? You can improve your risk for heart disease by eating better, exercising more, and getting more MUFAs.

Research on MUFAs and heart health is so compelling that a daily MUFA target is now part of the standard scientific protocol for preventing and managing cardiovascular disease (CVD) risk. The Therapeutic Lifestyle Changes plan, developed by the National Heart, Lung, and Blood Institute (a branch of the National Institutes of Health), is designed to reduce the risk of coronary heart disease.[12] It recommends a total fat intake of 25 to 35 percent of daily calories, with saturated fat making up no more than 7 percent of calories and MUFA composing up to 20 percent of total calories. Studies like the ones highlighted on the following pages have helped fuel these recommendations.

continued on page 36

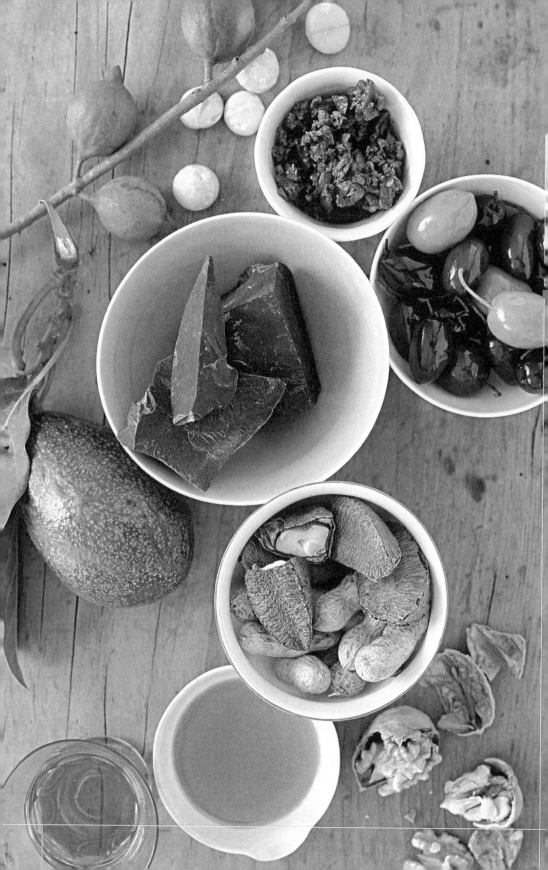

CHOOSE YOUR MUFA

These powerful MUFA–packed foods can help you live a long, healthy life while shrinking your gut at the same time. The best part is that these foods also provide a host of other beneficial nutrients.

1. Oils: The health benefits of the oils recommended by the Flat Belly Diet for Men (canola, safflower, sesame, soybean, walnut, flaxseed, sunflower, olive, and peanut) differ depending on the nut, seed, or fruit they were pressed from. Flaxseed and walnut oil are both rich sources of alpha-linolenic acid, which your body converts into omega-3 fatty acids. Extra-virgin olive oil has strong antibacterial properties and can even kill *H. pylori,* the bacterium that causes most peptic ulcers and some types of stomach cancer.[13] Olive oil also contains phyto-chemicals called polyphenols, which help prevent cardiovascular disease and cancer. Canola, sesame, sunflower, safflower, and soybean oils are all rich in vitamin E.

2. Olives: In addition to their MUFAs, olives are a good source of iron, vitamin E, copper (a mineral that protects your nerves, thyroid, and connective tissue), and fiber (which regulates your digestive system, helps control blood sugar levels, and manages blood cholesterol).

3. Nuts and Seeds: Like oils, the health benefits of the Flat Belly nuts and seeds are numerous and varied. Sun-flower seeds are a good source of linoleic acid. One recent study found that linoleic acid may lower the risk of developing high blood pressure.[14] The omega-3 fatty acids in walnuts have been linked to protection against inflammation, heart disease, asthma, and arthritis. Pistachios have been shown to help keep blood pressure down in stressful situations. Overall, nuts and seeds are good sources of many key nutrients, including protein, fiber, iron, zinc, magnesium, copper, B vitamins, and vitamin E.

4. Avocados: Avocados are packed with lutein, which may help maintain healthy eyes, as well as beta-sitosterol, which may help keep cholesterol down. Adding avocado has been shown to more than double the absorption of carotenoids, antioxidants linked to a lower risk of heart disease and macular degeneration.[15] Avocados are also rich in fiber, vitamin K (which helps clot blood), potassium (which regulates blood pressure), and heart-protective folate.

5. Dark Chocolate: Dark chocolate is rich in flavanols and proan-thocyanidins, both of which boost good HDL cholesterol levels. It also contains natural substances that help control insulin levels and lower blood pressure. Dark chocolate provides important minerals including copper, magnesium, potassium, calcium, and iron.

A recent analysis by researchers from Harvard University and the University of Oxford demonstrates a strong cardiovascular disease risk reduction in study participants who replace trans fat consumption with MUFAs.[16]

French scientists tested the effects of replacing some dietary carbohydrates with MUFAs without reducing calories. They found that the MUFA-rich diet produced better effects on blood triglyceride levels and other markers for CVD.[17]

Johns Hopkins University School of Medicine researchers compared the effects of three healthful diets, each with reduced saturated fat intake, on blood pressure and blood fat levels over 6 weeks, without allowing for weight loss.[18] The first diet was rich in carbohydrates, the second high in protein (with about half from plant sources), and the third high in MUFAs. They found that the protein and MUFA diets further lowered blood pressure, improved blood fat levels, and reduced the estimated risk of CVD.

Pennsylvania State University faculty compared the CVD risk profile of an average American diet to four cholesterol-lowering diets: an American Heart Association/National Cholesterol Education Program Step II diet and three high-MUFA diets.[19] The Step II diet and all of the high-MUFA diets lowered total cholesterol by 10 percent and LDL cholesterol by 14 percent. The MUFA diets also lowered triglyceride concentrations by 13 percent, while the Step II diet increased them by 11 percent. The MUFA diets preserved "good" HDL cholesterol, but the Step II diet lowered it by 4 percent.

University of Barcelona scientists examined the short-term effects of two Mediterranean diets versus a low-fat diet on markers of cardiovascular risk.[20] Compared with the low-fat diet, the mean changes in blood sugar, blood pressure, and cholesterol were significantly better in the MUFA-rich, olive oil–based Mediterranean diet and in the MUFA-rich, nut-based Mediterranean group.

MUFAs Reduce Metabolic Syndrome Risk

Metabolic syndrome in men can be diagnosed if they have three or more of the following: waist circumference greater than 40 inches, elevated triglyceride levels, low HDL cholesterol, elevated blood pressure, or elevated blood glucose.[21] This syndrome doubles a man's risk of having a stroke or dying from heart disease and increases his risk for type 2 diabetes. It's estimated that over 50 million Americans have this dreaded condition.

Researchers from the department of medicine at Columbia University in New York studied 52 men and 33 women with metabolic syndrome.[22] Over 7 weeks they were randomly assigned to either a typical American diet with 36 percent of calories from fat or two additional diets, in which 7 percent of the calories from saturated fat were replaced with either carbohydrates or MUFAs. The study found that LDL cholesterol was reduced with both of the lower-saturated-fat diets, but MUFAs protected HDL and lowered triglycerides, which were significantly higher with the high-carbohydrate diet.

MUFAs Ward Off Type 2 Diabetes

In type 2 diabetes (the most common form of diabetes), the body's cells cannot use glucose for energy, and as a result, this glucose collects in the blood. Over time, high blood glucose levels can damage the eyes, kidneys, nerves, and heart. About 21 million men have type 2 diabetes, or about 10 percent of the US population. Your risk for type 2 diabetes increases if you're overweight, inactive, or have a parent or sibling with type 2 diabetes.

A recent study conducted in Greece examined the effects of MUFAs on the blood vessels of people with type 2 diabetes. After just one meal of foods rich in saturated fat, participants' blood vessels were damaged. But a meal of MUFAs protected their blood vessels! (Damage to blood vessels causes many of the complications of type 2 diabetes, such as heart disease, kidney failure, or erectile dysfunction.)[23]

Spanish researchers studied the effects of three weight-maintenance diets on carbohydrate and fat metabolism and insulin levels in overweight subjects. The participants were randomly assigned to 28-day diets high in either saturated fats, MUFAs, or carbohydrates.[24] Fasting blood sugar levels fell on both the MUFA-rich and carb-rich diets, but the MUFA diet also improved insulin sensitivity and boosted HDL cholesterol levels.

At Indiana University, scientists treated type 2 diabetes patients with either a MUFA-rich weight-reducing diet or a low-fat, high-carbohydrate weight loss diet for 6 weeks.[25] Both groups lost pounds, but the MUFA group had a greater decrease in total cholesterol and triglyceride levels and a smaller drop in HDL cholesterol. These results were sustained even after the group was allowed to regain the weight.

MUFAs Lower Inflammation

Inflammation is basically our immune system's response to stress, injury, or illness. It's a known trigger for premature aging and chronic disease, including cancer, heart disease, and arthritis, but MUFAs are effective at quelling its "flames."

A Spanish study focused on a large group of men and women at high risk for cardiovascular disease.[26] It found that the consumption of particular Mediterranean foods, including MUFA-rich virgin olive oil and nuts, was associated with lower blood concentrations of inflammatory markers.

In an Italian study, the effect of a Mediterranean-style diet on inflammatory markers in patients with metabolic syndrome was studied.[27] Over 3 years, researchers randomly assigned nearly 200 men and women with metabolic syndrome to either a Mediterranean-style diet rich in whole grains, fruits, vegetables, and MUFA-rich nuts and olive oil or a "prudent" diet composed of 50 to 60 percent carbohydrate, 15 to 20 percent protein, and 30 percent or less fat (the old Dietary Guidelines standard). After 2 years, patients following the Mediterranean-style diet, who had consumed more total grams of MUFA and fiber per day, had a greater decrease in mean body weight. The high-MUFA diet also significantly reduced blood concentrations of inflammatory markers and decreased insulin resistance.

MUFAs Maintain Brain Health

The risk of Alzheimer's disease and other cognitive disorders increases with age. How can you help prevent this? More MUFAs!

Scientists in the Department of Geriatrics in the Center for Aging Brain at the University of Bari, Italy, set out to study the relationship between diet and age-related changes in cognitive functions. They looked at a sample of 5,632 people between the ages of 65 and 84 in eight regions of Italy.[28] They used a battery of standardized tests to assess cognitive function, selective attention, and memory and evaluated the subjects' diets. The study found that those with the highest percentage of calories from MUFAs had the greatest protection against cognitive decline.

Another Italian study, led by scientists at the same center's Memory Unit, investigated the role of diet in age-related cognitive decline (ARCD). They looked at an elderly population in southern Italy that consumed a typical Mediterranean diet and concluded that a high intake of MUFAs warded off ARCD.[29]

MUFAs Lower Prostate Cancer Risk

Prostate cancer is one of the most common types of cancer in men—it affects about one in six American men. Not only can it be life-threatening, but treatments for prostate cancer can cause erectile dysfunction and bladder control problems.

A New Zealand study used food frequency questionnaires to compare the diets of 317 men with prostate cancer to 480 men who didn't have the disease.[30] The results showed that increasing dietary levels of MUFA-rich vegetable oils, such as olive oil, peanut oil, and canola oil, was associated with a progressive reduction in prostate cancer risk. They also found that participants who consumed more than 5.5 milliliters of MUFA-rich vegetable oils per day had a high intake of vegetables, lycopene, vitamin E, selenium, and omega-3 fish oils, and eating these foods and nutrients may have added to the reduction in prostate cancer risk.

A Canadian study looked at the association between fat, prediagnostic energy, and vitamin A intake and survival rates among prostate cancer patients.[31] They examined 263 cases from the Canadian cities of Toronto and Vancouver. The participants provided their diet histories at diagnosis and were then followed to determine their survival from prostate cancer. The researchers found a strong significant inverse relationship between MUFA intake and the relative risk of dying from prostate cancer in both cities.

MUFAs Extend Your Life

We know you want to live a long, healthy life. Did you know that your wife or girlfriend is likely to outlive you by about 5 years? That's right, the current life expectancy for men in the United States is 75; for women, it's 80. One way you might be able to add extra years: MUFAs!

Several studies have looked at the link between MUFA intake and life expectancy. An 8½-year follow-up to the Italian Longitudinal Study on Aging investigated the possible role of MUFAs and other foods in protecting against all-causes mortality.[32] Among subjects without dementia between the ages of 65 and 84, scientists found that a higher MUFA intake was associated with increased survival, and there was no effect found in any other selected food group.

MUFAs Target Belly Fat

Men with belly fat are at greater risk for serious health problems (including heart disease, stroke, some types of cancer, and type 2 diabetes) than men without. And a Canadian study showed that visceral abdominal fat is a strong predictor of death in men.[33]

A 2007 study published in the journal *Diabetes Care* found that, compared to a diet high in carbohydrates or saturated fats at the same calorie level, a MUFA-rich diet prevented "central body fat distribution"— in other words, if you eat a MUFA-rich diet, you're less likely to accumulate visceral fat and therefore less likely to develop many of the diseases listed above.[34]

MESSAGE FROM MILTON

"My Favorite MUFA"

On any given day my meals include a vegetable oil of some sort, nuts, and dark chocolate squares. My favorite type of cuisine, however, is Mexican and Tex-Mex. Anything hot and spicy, and I'm there. So, naturally, avocado and guacamole are my go-to MUFAs. And the hotter, the better! In fact, I grow jalapeños in my garden, and each summer I look forward to throwing a couple diced peppers into my homemade guacamole. It's a MUFA with a kick.

Australian researchers randomly assigned overweight men to various 4-week diets with the same calorie level but different amounts of saturated, monounsaturated, and polyunsaturated fat. The MUFA-rich diet resulted in lower total body weight and body fat. The authors concluded that a high-MUFA diet can induce a significant loss of body weight and fat mass without a change in total calorie or fat intake.

Another Australian study compared post-meal body fat burning rates after two breakfasts: one with saturated fat from cream and one with MUFA from olive oil.[35] The MUFA group had a significantly higher fat-burning rate in the 5 hours after breakfast, particularly in the subjects with greater abdominal fat.

The Other Spare Tire Solution: Attitude

ULTIMATELY, THE FLAT BELLY DIET FOR MEN isn't just about the food, though delicious food never hurts! But before we get to the actual eating plan, I want to emphasize the one factor that will be key to whether you actually lose your gut—and that's your state of mind. Your stress levels, how you handle everyday things like anger and boredom, and even what runs through your mind when you catch a glimpse of your gut can all play a role in how and what you eat. It can even help determine how and where you put on weight. It's true; your mental state can actually impact the size of your paunch.

In the next chapter, we'll explore some common challenges that can stand in the way of men trying to lose that spare tire. We'll also reveal the simple secrets to succeeding on the Flat Belly Diet for Men.

The Danger of Skipping Meals

It doesn't pay to try to dip below the 2,000-calories-a-day mark. Believe me, I understand the temptation. We've all been led to believe that the fewer calories we ingest, the faster we'll lose weight. But weight loss isn't quite that simple. If you drastically cut down on the amount of food you eat for any extended time, your body's natural response is to slow things down to conserve fat. If you're looking for six-pack abs, that "starvation response" is the last thing you need.

Here's what happens: If you take in too few calories, your body starts breaking down muscle tissue to use for fuel. That muscle loss can drastically affect your metabolism, often for a long time. The reason is simple: Muscle is metabolically active tissue that requires a certain number of calories each day to maintain itself, whether or not it's in use. So the more muscle you have, the more calories you burn. As your muscle mass drops, so does your body's need for calories to sustain it. Let's say a dieter on a too-strict plan loses 15 pounds, 10 pounds of which is fat and 5 pounds of which is muscle. Let's also assume that every pound of muscle burns about 50 calories a day. With this muscle tissue gone, the dieter must now consume 250 (5 times 50) fewer calories a day to maintain his 15-pound weight loss. Of course, most dieters don't stick to the strict routine for long. They return to their pre-diet eating habits. And that's what puts them at risk of regaining all their lost weight—and then some more.

READ A FLAT BELLY
SUCCESS
STORY

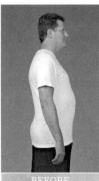

BEFORE

Alan Musselman

AGE: 48

POUNDS LOST:

19.2

IN 32 DAYS

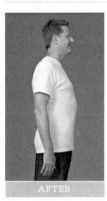

AFTER

ALL-OVER INCHES LOST:

8.5

3.5 FROM THE WAIST

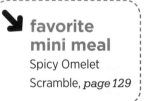

↘ **favorite mini meal**
Spicy Omelet
Scramble, *page 129*

"It's the beers that got me here!" exclaimed Alan, pointing vigorously at his "before" picture. "I spent a lot of calories on alcohol, and, well, I had the beer belly to show for it." Now, 19.2 pounds lighter and 8.5 inches smaller, Alan, a 48-year-old financial officer from Pennsylvania, is healthier, happier, and wearing a much smaller pants size!

His girlfriend, Ginger Horsford, recalls, "He was walking from the living room to the kitchen one night, and boom, down his pants went!"

Alan adds, "I have gotten used to people making comments about my weight loss and the fact that my belly no longer sticks out."

Before Alan started the Flat Belly Diet for Men, Alan and Ginger spent time revamping their pantry, stocking up on ingredients, and getting organized. "We wanted to ensure we were both prepared with the right foods so everything could be streamlined," says Alan. And it worked. He lost an impressive 4 pounds in the 4 days of the Flat Abs Kickstart and continued to drop weight throughout the Four-Week MUFA Meal Plan.

A lover of all things spicy, Alan enjoyed the Fire Water and used hot sauce in most of the Four-Week MUFA Meal Plan recipes—and continued to drop pounds. The bit of heat served as a reminder that he was eating better and doing something healthy for himself. "I feel better and look better than I have in years," Alan says. "I feel younger. I look forward to getting on the scale instead of hiding from it."

An avid runner, Alan found his weight loss improved not only his racing times, but also his attitude. "With my new body and positive outlook, I can't wait to run these days. I am running without pain and my running times are faster. At the last race with my running buddy Don, I actually felt like a college student running on the cross-country team. I even passed him—something I haven't done in years! Thank you, Flat Belly Diet for Men for making my running (and my life!) fun again!"

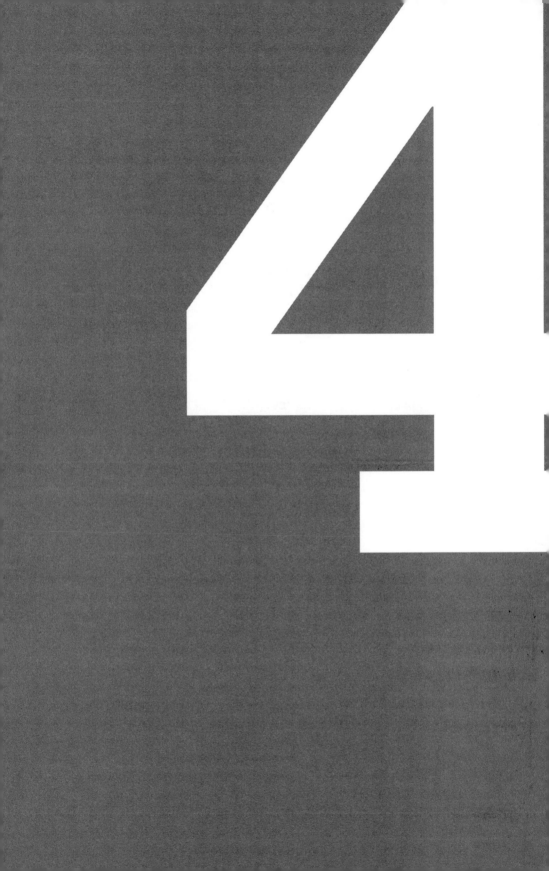

THE CHALLENGES
OF WEIGHT
LOSS

WANT IN ON a secret? The true key to successfully eliminating your paunch is your state of mind. It's true. The relationship between the mind and body is a scientifically solid one. Understanding how they work together will make the difference between whether or not you reach your weight loss goal—or really any lifestyle goal. Why? Consider the impact your attitude can have on what you eat, how much you eat, and when you eat it.

You know the stereotype: A woman turns to a pint of ice cream when she isn't feeling great about herself. But just because there aren't many stereotypes like that for men, it doesn't mean that having a spare tire is a boost to a guy's self-esteem! It's exactly the opposite—guys also are affected by how they look. And stereotypes or no, there's always that pint of beer waiting for a guy to drown his sorrows.

Truly, we can't emphasize the mind-body connection enough. Milton has a patient in his private practice who was able to boost his weight loss by simply practicing mindful eating. This patient has idiopathic gastroparesis, a condition where the stomach won't empty normally. The cause is unknown, and eating fast and mindlessly makes the problem worse. For several years this patient would eat large portions quickly and then end up sick and throwing up in the bathroom every night. Gradually reducing the speed of eating and trying to put his fork down more frequently helped Milton's patient eat less, minimize some of the complications from gastroparesis, and lose 10 pounds in a month.

Many other obstacles can stand in the way of your tighter abs, whether it's rising stress levels, regularly grabbing fast food on the go, your weekly poker night, or scarfing down junk food whenever boredom hits. We at *Prevention* magazine know from years of talking to men (and their wives, girlfriends, and significant others) that attitude, thoughts, habits, and practically everything mind-related can influence what foods you choose to eat and the way you eat them. That's why the Flat Belly Diet for Men is about engaging your mind as much as your taste buds. Getting your brain on board is the first step to washboard abs!

Get in the Game

HERE'S SOMETHING TO CONSIDER: Hunger actually starts in your brain, not in your stomach. Physiologically speaking, your appetite is controlled by biochemical signals that tell your brain that you're hungry and need to eat or are satisfied and can stop. While men and women gain weight due to different stressors, everyone knows how to override their brain signals. Nowadays, we eat not only when we're hungry, but also when we're bored, happy, anxious, sad . . . you get the picture. Really, there's usually no excuse needed to overindulge in your favorite food or beverage, but both men and women are guilty of doing it.

To get a handle on this behavior, you first must understand why you do it. For one thing, many of us have been conditioned to believe that food makes you feel better (remember getting a lollipop after a shot at the doctor's?). And it does—at least in the short term. As adults, many of us turn to food to combat stress and don't hesitate to snack when we're feeling bored, anxious, or even angry.

For many of us, years spent addressing everything but an empty stomach with food means we have to relearn what actual hunger feels like. It may sound strange, but many people have forgotten what it feels like to be hungry, even though the line between emotional and true hunger is pretty clear-cut. Researchers at the University of Texas Counseling and Mental Health Center have identified five ways to distinguish between the two:[1]

"Emotional," or "bogus," hunger comes on suddenly, while physical hunger is gradual.

Physical hunger is felt below the neck (think growling stomach), while emotional hunger is felt above the neck (like a sudden craving for pizza).

When only a certain food—say a burger or nachos—will satisfy you, your "hunger" is born of emotion. When your body requires fuel, you're more open to food options.

Bogus hunger wants to be satisfied instantly. Physical hunger can wait.

Bogus hunger leaves guilt in its wake. Physical hunger doesn't.

Once you start paying attention to these signals, you'll have an easier time distinguishing a bogus need for food from a physical one. The next time a craving strikes, try this: Tune out the signals coming from the neck up. Are you really physically hungry?

The way to really beat bogus eating, though, is to develop some hard-hitting effective strategies. While seeking out distractions or a good time provides some relief, it's not the solution. Here's an example: If you're stressed out and craving a burger and fries, watching a ball game on TV may distract you for a while, but it's not likely to eliminate the stress. Instead, acknowledge that you're feeling stressed out and then try to figure out what is really going on. Confronting the stress (or boredom, sadness, anger, or other feeling) immediately rather than avoiding it is the best way to beat that desire to chow down on wings or gulp beer. Admit how you feel, take back control, and put down that beer!

Of course, this is easier said than done, but before we delve into the tools and tips you need to beat bogus eating, let's take a look at what all this stress is doing to you.

Scrutinizing the Stress Effect

UNFORTUNATELY, STRESS IS ALL too common in today's fast-paced world. Too much stress can start fueling weight gain, and many male guts have stress to blame. But stress isn't just one thing. When scientists study stress, they always differentiate between two types: acute, or short-term, and chronic, or long-term. Not sure of the difference? An example of chronic stress could be if you're constantly struggling to make ends meet. Acute stress could be something as simple as being late for a meeting or as serious as almost getting into a car accident.

The Biology of Acute Stress

Back in the Stone Age, cavemen's very survival depended on their ability to respond instantly to short-term stresses like being chased by predators. Today,

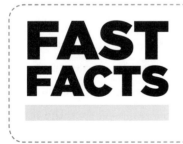

Certain foods can help decrease stress. A survey that asked participants to track the food-mood connection found that increasing consumption of water, vegetables, fruits, fish, nuts, and whole grains and decreasing intake of sugar, caffeine, and alcohol had a dramatic stress-reducing impact.[2]

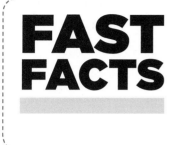

we're still equipped with a hair-trigger mechanism that overrides our rational minds in an emergency or when we feel threatened. We call this the fight-or-flight response, and it's no different if the stressor is a ravenous beast or an impatient boss. Here's how it works.

Stress responses start in the nervous system. The central nervous system (CNS) responds to orders from the conscious mind, while the autonomic nervous system (ANS) functions independently. If you decide, for example, to take a picture of a friend with your cell phone, the CNS puts into play all the actions needed to complete the task, from having the idea to snapping the shutter. Meanwhile, you will continue to breathe (without having to think about it), and your body will continue to go on digesting food, pumping blood, and fending off harmful bacteria. Your ANS governs these functions, operating without a single conscious thought or action on your part.

There are two branches within the ANS: the sympathetic nervous system (SNS) and the parasympathetic nervous system (PNS). The first revs you up, and the second calms you down. Say, for example, you're crossing a busy intersection and see a zooming bus coming toward you. You don't consciously demand that your heart pump faster and deliver more blood to your muscles so they can react with more force to get you out of the way; you just naturally jump onto the curb. In that mere millisecond, your brain perceives the threat and kicks the SNS into high gear. Then the rest of your body kicks in. Here's what happens.

▪ The hypothalamus in the brain sends a message to your adrenal glands near your kidneys, which pump out the hormones adrenaline and cortisol (more on this later).

▪ Adrenaline increases your heartbeat to twice its normal speed, sending extra blood to the brain, as well as to the major muscles in your arms and legs. This makes you better able to dodge that zooming bus.

▪ Your memory gets sharper.

▪ Your immune system goes on alert in case it's needed to fight infection from an impending wound.

▪ Your arteries narrow, so you'll lose less blood if you get injured. Narrowed arteries cause an increase in blood pressure.

▪ Your pupils dilate and your vision becomes more acute.

Signs of Chronic Stress

The following are some of the most common signs that you may be suffering from chronic stress. Of course, if you experience more severe symptoms, your depressed mood lasts for more than 2 weeks or is seriously interfering with your daily activities, or if you find your-self treating your stress with drugs or alcohol, please see your doctor or a therapist.

Headaches

Muscular tension

Tightness in your chest and a feeling that you can't catch your breath

Frequent upset stomach, indigestion, trapped wind, diarrhea, or appetite changes

Frequent illness

Hives or skin rashes

Tooth grinding

Feeling faint or dizzy

Ringing in the ears

Low sex drive

Sleep disturbance: either insomnia or hypersomnia (sleeping too much)

Mental or physical fatigue

Feeling overly nervous, sad, irritable, or angry

Having problems at work or in your normal relationships

Apathy (lack of interest, motivation, or energy)

- Your digestive system slows down.
- Insulin production ramps up, overriding signals from adrenaline to burn fat, and encourages the body to store it in anticipation of future needs.

Pretty amazing, right? All this happens to safely get you out of that barreling bus's way—and, in the Stone Age, to enable our ancestors to dodge that hungry saber-toothed tiger intent on landing its next meal. When the immediate threat is over, so is the short-term stress. That's when the PNS steps in, releasing calming hormones that help your body return to equilibrium.

The Consequences of Chronic Stress

Unlike acute stress, which has a beginning and an end, chronic stress is ongoing. This is what makes chronic stress dangerous. When your job is on shaky ground, your marriage hits a rough patch, your bank account is dwindling, your aging parents suddenly need a lot more care—or all of these things happen at once!—that is chronic stress. (It may seem counterintuitive, but chronic stress can also result from positive things! While landing a new job, getting married, or having a baby is each an exciting life event, they're also different than what you're used to, and so they can cause stress.)

The problem is your body still reacts as if these stresses were acute, yet—and here's the important distinction—there's no calming period. The SNS just keeps doing its stuff, keeping you in a state of heightened physiological arousal as if your very life were being threatened all the time, every day. The more your body's stress response system is activated, the harder it is to switch off. And that's a major concern, given that anywhere from 60 to 90 percent of illness is stress-related.

Here's how the stress/health connection works: The adrenal glands secrete an abundance of the hormone cortisol during times of stress. Under normal circumstances, cortisol's role is to regulate blood pressure, cardiovascular function, and metabolism. Your body can easily handle the occasional burst of cortisol when it's triggered by an acute or high-stress moment. But when stress is chronic, causing a steady stream of cortisol to flow into your bloodstream, that's when things start to go bad.

Too much cortisol weakens your immune system, puts your heart into overdrive, and raises your blood pressure. A consistently high level of circulating stress hormones adversely affects brain function as well, especially memory. Not only that, but excessive cortisol can interfere with "feel good" neurotransmitters, such as dopamine and serotonin, making you more vulnerable to depression. Basically, nothing good can come healthwise from chronic stress.

Simple Stress-Fighters

SINCE YOUR SOURCES OF STRESS are personal, so should be the strategies you use to counteract their day-to-day effects. Steve and I go for regular exercise, watching mindless TV, or playing a routing game of tag or hide-and-seek with our girls. Some men who've written to *Prevention* magazine tell me how they hang out with their buddies regularly to unwind, while others get focus and perspective by shooting hoops or playing the drums. And Milton likes to catch

Let's Talk about Sex

Sex—it's everyone's favorite stress reducer, but as you probably know, it can also be a cause of stress, too. Stress can cause sexual dysfunction: If a guy gets fired, he may not feel like jumping into bed immediately. But the reverse is also true: If things aren't going well in the bedroom, that can cause stress. Add it up, and a guy can be caught in a sex-free cycle! Just one more reason to follow the advice in this chapter about methods to de-stress! (And one more reason to follow the Flat Belly Diet for Men: Without that spare tire, you'll most likely feel sexier, and your libido will most likely improve. Then you'll want to use sex as a stress reducer as often as possible!)

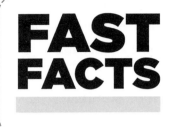

up on the day's entertainment news, take his dog Mac for a walk, and watch *Saturday Night Live* clips online.

Though every man has his own tactics to counter stress, researchers have determined that certain behaviors can be helpful in allowing guys to manage their busy lives, cope with anxiety, and just be happier overall. In the process, these strategies can help minimize a stress-induced gut, too. Use this list like a tool kit. The more tools you use, the more you—and your belly—will benefit.

1. GET A CLUE. What causes you to be stressed out constantly? As found by the Harvard researchers in a study discussed on page 51, for men, it's most likely problems at work. Take note of these things and then, when possible, sidestep them. When you are on edge, you may find yourself leaning on your car horn, forgetting important appointments, or even yelling at your kids. But if you think about what's bothering you—really bothering you—you'll most likely discover it's not your children or the traffic. It's that you've maxed out what I call your "stress reserves." When this happens, remove yourself from the scene and break the stress cycle. Just walk away. Literally. Go around the block or into the next room. If that is impossible, simply close your eyes, count to 10, and breathe deeply. Those few moments might give you a chance to process strong emotions before they overwhelm you. You should also feel better physically almost immediately. Of course, if you experience severe symptoms for extended times, please see your doctor or a therapist.

2. GET ENOUGH REST. At the turn of the 20th century, the average American typically slept about 9 hours a night. Can you imagine? These days most of us are lucky to get 7 hours. And while you might think it's macho to attempt to get by on just a few hours of sleep, this is a big mistake. I've known executive power players (CEOs, stock brokers, etc.) who boast about getting by on just 3 hours of sleep a night. They are also overweight, stressed out, and unhealthy. Ummm, way to go?

Lack of sleep doesn't just lead to fatigue; it can also make you stressed—and fat. Consistently depriving yourself of rest puts your body under a constant level of elevated stress. It also results in reduced levels of leptin, a protein that regulates body fat and increases ghrelin, which stimulates appetite. The result? Your body stores fat, your metabolism slows, and you want to eat more. Downtime is necessary for your body to revitalize and replenish its reserves. This is especially true for anyone trying to drop pounds. Why? It's much harder to summon the physical energy and mental focus to stick to any diet or exercise plan if you're sleep deprived. So if you do nothing else on this list, make sure you get a good night's sleep.

The following ideas can help you get your ZZZs:

■ **GO DARK.** Any light will signal the brain to wake up, especially "blue light" from your cell phone and your clock's digital display. So dim your clock and remove lighted devices from your bedroom.

Walk for Deep Sleep

A little walking goes a long way toward getting a sound night's sleep. When researchers studied more than 700 men and women, they found that those who walked at least six blocks a day at a moderate pace were one-third less likely to have sleeping problems than those who walked shorter distances. Those who walked at a brisker pace were most likely of all to enjoy sound sleep.[5] Other studies show that a regular walking program is as effective at improving sleep as medication.

■ **STAY ON SCHEDULE.** People who follow regular daily routines report fewer sleep problems than those with more unpredictable lifestyles, according to a study from the University of Pittsburgh Medical Center. Recurring time cues will synchronize your body rhythms and sleep-wake cycles, explains Lawrence Epstein, MD, of Harvard Medical School, a renowned expert on insomnia.[6]

■ **SLIP ON SOME SOCKS.** Yes, socks. The instant warmth provided by socks widens blood vessels and allows your body to transfer heat from its core to the extremities, cooling you slightly. This induces sleep, says Phyllis Zee, PhD, director of sleep disorders at Northwestern University's Feinberg School of Medicine.[7]

3. GET PHYSICAL. Studies show that even 10 minutes of physical activity will help reduce cortisol levels in the bloodstream. Exercise does this by changing your body's biochemistry. It triggers the brain to produce beta-endorphins, chemicals that calm you down, regulate your stress hormones, and make you feel good. So the next time you feel your blood pressure rising, head for the door and take a bike ride or a quick walk around the block. A little physical activity may not solve the problem at hand, but it will certainly help you cope with it.

But don't overdo it! The last thing you want to do is add a pulled muscle or stress fracture to your stressful life. If you're not used to exercising, start slowly, and if you're already a gym rat, increase your exercise routine gradually.

4. GET CONNECTED. Guys may be less likely than women to reach out when they are stressed out, but doing so can be really beneficial. Talking or interacting with others can defuse your feelings of tension. Studies have shown that even just being in someone's company—without saying a word—helps alleviate stress. It also promotes good health. Research shows that people who maintain personal and community connections have better health than those who don't. But you don't have to sit down and have a heart-to-heart with your buddies whenever you're feeling anxious. Stress-reducing connections can be made simply by shooting hoops with the guys, chatting with your bartender, connecting with your peeps online through social networking sites, or (most men's favorite stress reducer) having sex with your partner. Socializing online certainly shouldn't replace face-to-face interactions, but social networking sites can also bring together like-minded people for conversation, collaboration, and information exchange, and provide an excellent opportunity for men to "get connected."

5. GET A NEW ATTITUDE. Whenever you catch yourself thinking, "I'll never get this report done," or, "I don't make enough money to support my family," stop yourself and change your thinking. Instead, replay the thought with an upbeat spin: "I will do my best to meet this deadline," and, "I'm doing everything I can for my family." I know, I know—you feel silly forcing yourself to think these thoughts. But believe me, it will help you feel more in control of your life and boost your confidence. And by now we know how vital these things are to eliminating that gut! When you feel overwhelmed, you can remind yourself that following the Flat Belly Diet for Men is something good you're doing for yourself!

6. PUT IT ON THE CALENDAR. Now that you've made your health an important priority, it's time to put you—and your gut—into action. So how about starting with 5 minutes a day to make a plan? Spending just a few minutes each

Not All Stress Is Harmful

We've been talking all about how you can de-stress your life, but you actually do need *some* stress to be happy—otherwise you'd be so bored you'd be stressed out! A study conducted at a Volvo car factory in Sweden showed that job satisfaction improved and workers' blood pressures dropped when they were switched from a repetitive, assembly-line workplace to a team-based, more flexible workplace.[8]

Drinking alcohol while on the Flat Belly Diet for Men is your decision. When I counsel clients individually, I tell them that the current dietary guidelines recommend if you don't drink, there's no reason to start. And you may wonder, "What about all the benefits to drinking?"

We have *some* evidence showing that moderate alcohol consumption might reduce the risk of heart disease; however, not every drinker responds favorably. It's easy to overdo alcohol. Excessive drinking is associated with liver disease, high blood pressure, cancers of the upper gastrointestinal tract, stroke, injuries, and violence.

That said, most men do consume alcohol. So if you already drink, practice moderation, meaning up to two drinks per day. (One drink equals 12 ounces of regular beer, 5 ounces of wine, or 1.5 ounces—one shot—of 80-proof distilled spirits.) Each of these contains around 100 calories, so to stay on track with the Flat Belly Diet for Men, you'll need to balance out those calories. If you plan to have one drink, you can either burn 100 extra calories by exercising or shave 25 calories from each of your four meals—or 50 each from two. Taking 100 calories out of a single 400-calorie meal can leave you feeling too hungry, and since alcohol is an appetite stimulant, that could be a recipe for overeating.

day to schedule your exercise, strategize your meals, or think about your ultimate goal will not only put your mind in the game, it will give you the time to formulate a plan to do so. Would you miss a work meeting? Or be late for a client call or appointment? Treat your weight loss like a job, and you're sure to see results.

Conquering Other Weight-Loss Challenges

STRESS AND ANXIETY aren't the only things that can fuel a guy's gut, unfortunately. There are many other obstacles that stand between a man and his six-pack abs. It's easy to fall into any of these traps and often hard to escape. The good news is that with our easy tips, you can learn to make better everyday decisions and combat weight gain all over your body—including in your belly.

Here are some common weight-boosting scenarios men face and some simple ways to overcome them.

Beers and the boys. Okay, male bonding is important; no one would deny that. It can help combat stress and allow you to feel more connected to your buddies. Unfortunately, these social outings often involve gut-unfriendly activities, like pounding back numerous beers and eating fried and fast foods. Though beer alone isn't to blame for a beer gut, drinking too much of any alcohol can cause you to gain belly fat—and when you drink, you also tend to eat more.[9] To minimize the negative impact of guys' night out, try eating one of the Flat Belly Diet for Men dinners before heading out to meet

Hunt for MUFAs

Eating away from home is a part of life. Whether for convenience, celebrations, or family nights out, restaurant dining is here to stay. If, like many men, you tend to frequent the same restaurants over and over, go online or ask for in-house nutrition brochures, and find MUFAs and healthy picks at your favorite joints. Reviewing menus in advance allows you to pick foods and remain within your caloric budget. I have my clients ask restaurants to fax menus to me so we can review them together and select healthier, calorie-conscious choices. Be sure you eat normally throughout the day. Some of my clients tried to skip breakfast and lunch so they could eat more at their restaurant dinner. But that's certainly a recipe for overeating. Planning ahead sets you up for success so you don't arrive starved with inhibitions totally turned off. Who can think clearly with an empty stomach screaming "feed me!"? Eating normally throughout the day puts you in a good place mentally. Apart from providing yourself balanced nutrition during the day, you may want to have a small snack of about 100 to 200 calories before you go. This helps ensure you don't binge eat later on. Lastly, try to steer clear of heavy sauces, creams, and fried foods.

the boys, so you'll be less tempted to indulge later. Also, stick to two beers or any other drinks for the night so you limit the number of calories consumed. And consider how the calories from the beer fit into your overall calorie strategy (see "What about Alcohol?"). You might also suggest taking guys' night out of the bar, and perhaps organize a poker night. Better yet, kick the activity into high gear and head out for a day of hiking, fishing, snowboarding, or golf.

Sedentary work and play. Many of you guys work 9-to-5 desk jobs, so most of your waking hours are spent sitting. This can not only be detrimental to your health, it can also result in a spare tire. While quitting your job is likely not an option, there are things you can do at work to combat the weight gain that comes with being sedentary. For example:

 Use the stairs instead of the elevator when going to and from your office, and be sure to park your car far away from the building's front door so you can squeeze in some extra walking time. Better yet, bike or walk to work.

 Take frequent breaks to stretch and walk around the office or outside.

 Eat a proper breakfast and lunch to ward off cravings during the day. For when those hunger or boredom pangs do hit, make sure your desk is stocked with MUFA-rich snacks so you're not tempted to eat everything in sight.

 Head to the gym over your lunch break if there's one in your office building or close by.

And what about when you get home from work? Time in front of the television, video games, or computer is also sedentary. And you may be snacking while sitting. Try to limit your screen time to 1 to 2 hours a night. With the rest of your time, surprise your wife or girlfriend by cooking dinner, meet the guys for a game of basketball, or take the dog for a walk.

Sporting events and other activities. Whether you're at a game, the movies, or a carnival, food options at events aren't usually very gut-friendly (or cheap, for that matter). Those pretzels, hot dogs, and fries can wreak havoc on your gut, not to mention those super-sized sodas and beers. While going to a game once in a while and indulging isn't going to cause any permanent belly damage, being a frequent spectator can make you more spare-tire prone.

 Control your hunger. Have a Flat Belly meal or snack before going to an event, and you'll be a lot less likely to overindulge in the not-so-healthy options.

 Pick wisely. Items that are battered or crispy tend to be fried and full of calories, while choices that are grilled, baked, or roasted are usually healthier and lower in calories. The smaller the size you order, the better.

 Limit alcohol. The calories in beer (and all other alcoholic drinks) are just as harmful as the calories in hot dogs, fries, and buttery popcorn. Have just one or two drinks, period.

 Implement damage control. If you fall off the good-for-you bandwagon (have a few too many beers, wings, or burgers, for example), don't get frustrated and throw in the Flat Belly towel. Instead, increase your activity over the next several days to minimize the damage.

Globetrotting. Whether traveling for business or pleasure, many men fall off the health wagon when they're on the road. It's easy for your health and belly-reducing routine to go awry, thanks to widely available fast food, lack of time, and being in unfamiliar territory. Unfortunately, taking a break from your health routine, especially if it's a permanent one, can be detrimental for your paunch. Here are some ideas to stay on track.

 Pack and carry around your own MUFA-rich, healthy snacks, such as nuts. This way you won't be tempted to pick up a bag of chips or scarf down some cookies when the munchies hit.

 Research restaurants and fast-food joints in advance to determine which ones are most likely to provide healthier, gut-fighting options. Some places will list their menus online or you can call a restaurant in advance. Better yet, get a hotel room with a kitchen so you can prepare some meals on your own.

Expense account eating can be dangerous for your belly. You may think, "Well, the company's picking up the tab, so I'll go for the fried appetizer, huge steak, and the bottle of wine," but you're only hurting yourself. Skip the greasy appetizer in favor of a salad, order a smaller steak (or only eat half of what you're served), and enjoy a glass or two of wine.

Use the hotel's gym or fitness room to maintain your workout routine. If your hotel doesn't have a fitness center, ask the front desk about what's available for travelers who want to exercise. If gyms aren't your thing, go for a walk or a jog instead—and do some exploring at the same time.

Family matters. Trying to lose weight if your family or partner is not backing you up is tough. Try this: Start by letting your loved ones know your plan to improve your health and your diet. Share your copy of the *Flat Belly Diet! for Men* with them. Inform them about the tasty MUFAs and the delicious Flat Belly meals and recipes, and invite them to take part in the food shopping and preparation. Ask them to remove temptation and keep junk food out of the house (and no, you really don't need junk food "just for the kids"). Invite them to join you in your quest to make healthier choices. Even if your loved ones don't need to lose weight, anytime is a good time to live healthier. Make your better-for-you lifestyle a family affair and you'll not only gain support and kitchen help, you'll teach the people you love how to better take care of themselves. It's a Flat Belly win-win!

Armed and Ready for Tight Abs

THE SCIENTIFIC UNDERPINNINGS of both bogus eating and the body's physiological response to stress should now be clear. You're also equipped with seven simple stress-busters, as well as easy ways to handle weight-boosting scenarios that men often find themselves in. By understanding this mind-body connection and equipping yourself with these gut-busting tools, you're finally ready to start the first part of the Flat Belly Diet for Men eating plan. The Four-Day Flat Abs Kickstart will make full use of all your newfound knowledge and start you down the road to a flatter gut!

Stop Wasting Time

A little time management can go a long way to remedy stress. Keep in mind: Time management isn't necessarily about doing more—it's about doing more of the things you want to do. Try tracking your time for a day or two to find out where your time is really going.

Set up a daily spreadsheet on your computer or in a notebook, broken into 15-minute blocks. Track what you do in each block of time from when you wake up to when you go to bed, and evaluate each day. Seeing how you actually spend your time throughout the day may help you determine how you can make changes that reduce your stress and improve your ability to fit in healthy meals, more physical activity, or a little downtime.

MESSAGE FROM MILTON

"Don't Become a Slave to the Scale"

I've seen countless patients in my practice over the years, most of whom wanted to lose weight. Their success (or failure) in their quest was usually dependent on their state of mind. I'd hear something like this from many patients struggling to lose weight: "What's fun or exciting or easy about losing weight? Not much. There's just so much pressure!"

On the other hand, when patients were changing their diets to feel better, have more energy, and improve their lives, the weight loss was almost a beneficial side effect.

It's easy to overemphasize body weight. Step back and take it all in. Tell yourself that your goal is to improve your health. To add a MUFA to each meal. To eat more frequently throughout the day. To eat reasonable portions. And the weight will come off . . . naturally.

READ A FLAT BELLY
SUCCESS
STORY

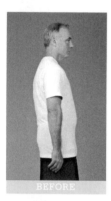

BEFORE

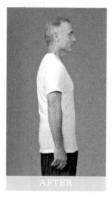

AFTER

John Rau

AGE: 55

POUNDS LOST:

17.2

IN 32 DAYS

ALL-OVER
INCHES LOST:

9.75

4 FROM
THE WAIST

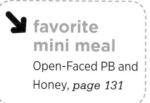

favorite mini meal
Open-Faced PB and Honey, *page 131*

"Eating smaller meals throughout the day was my key to success," explains John, a 55-year-old software developer from Long Island, New York. "I truly love food—all cuisines and dishes—and I enjoy cooking. I also use food as a comforter and stress reliever." In the past, John would sometimes go hours between meals, so he was starving by the time he sat down to eat—hence, he overate and packed on the pounds. But with the Flat Belly Diet, "I never got overly hungry."

John's weight loss battle started soon after high school, and his weight fluctuated dramatically over the years, culminating in an all-time high of 223 pounds. "I would use a combination of severe calorie reduction and vigorous exercise to lose the weight. Conversely, I then stuffed my face because I was starving and inevitably gained the weight back." From a juice-only diet, to diet pills, and more, John would lose some weight, only to eventually pack it back on.

Even during his ups and downs with weight, John was always active. "Whether it was tennis, weight lifting, running marathons, or working out on the cross trainer, I kept busy with exercises I enjoyed." His downfall, though, was always the food. But the Flat Belly Diet for Men changed all that!

"With this plan, I learned how to cook with less fat and with healthier ingredients and still have delicious meals. The food tastes great!" Not missing the extra calories from fat-laden dishes, John says that he and his wife of 24 years, Nancy, applied Flat Belly Diet for Men cooking techniques to some of their favorite recipes. "We tweaked recipes that we had been making for years. By adding less fat, my dishes became lighter and healthier while remaining just as satisfying." John also attributes some of his success to drinking Fire Water. "I felt like it gave my metabolism a boost." The Fire Water also helped ensure John stayed hydrated during all of his exercise. With more than 17 pounds gone and just a few to go before reaching his final weight goal of 180, John is quite pleased with himself—and he should be!

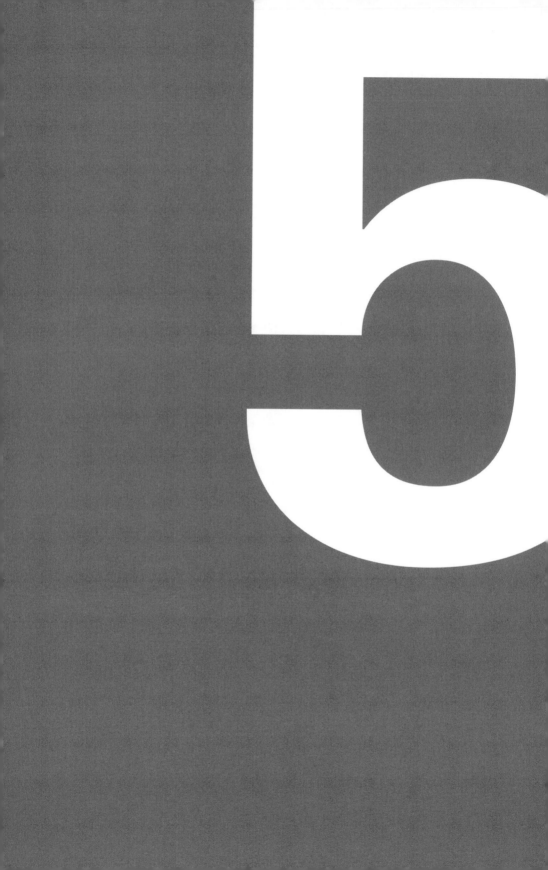

THE FOUR-DAY
FLAT ABS
KICKSTART

OKAY GUYS, IT'S time to kick your weight loss into high gear! The Flat Abs Kickstart is designed to flush out fluids, boost your metabolism, and jumpstart your weight loss by picking just the right amount of digestion-friendly foods and drinks. Just like a professional athlete preparing to "make weight" in his weight class, you'll be shedding water and dropping pounds—fast! In just 4 days, you'll lose several pounds and inches, which will start a cascade of motivation and energy that will immediately set you up for success on the rest of the plan.

How do I know? Because Milton and I tested the entire Flat Belly Diet for Men plan—including the Kickstart—on men just like you. You're reading their stories throughout this book. More than half of our test panel lost around 4 pounds and 3 inches from their bellies during the Kickstart period. There's nothing more satisfying when you're starting a new eating plan than being able to see—almost immediately—your trousers getting looser and your muscles getting more defined. It inspires commitment and a desire to succeed. And that's what I want you to get out of this book more than anything else: success.

The Four-Day Flat Abs Kickstart has been created for the very specific purpose of eliminating gas and excess water so you will quickly feel and look lighter. Therefore, you won't be getting a "MUFA at every meal" until the Four-Week MUFA Meal Plan, when you start concentrating on visceral belly fat. But don't worry: This is not a wacky detox plan. This isn't even a very stringent diet. You'll be eating whole fruits, vegetables, and grains and drinking fresh, naturally flavored water. In other words, you'll be eating real food. It's what you won't be eating and drinking and doing that really makes the Kickstart so effective. To see how it works, I think it helps to first understand your digestive system.

Digestion: The Basics

YOUR GASTROINTESTINAL (GI) tract is about 35 feet long from top to bottom. Read that again: 35 feet long! That's about six of you, lying end to end. And it's all coiled up inside your torso (along with most of your major organs and, yes, belly fat). That's why, when your GI tract is irritated or in any way dysfunctional, it greatly impacts how you feel overall. But before we talk about potential problems, let's go over the basics.

The primary role of your GI tract is to extract essential nutrients like carbohydrates, proteins, fats, vitamins, minerals, and water from the food you eat and the beverages you drink. These nutrients are transported through the walls of the small and large intestines into the bloodstream, where they're then distributed to wherever they're needed. For instance, when you eat a hamburger, your GI tract breaks it down into bits of carbohydrate (the bread), protein (the hamburger meat), fat (the mayo), fiber (the bread), and all sorts of

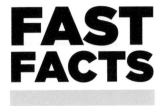

FAST FACTS

The word *metabolism* refers to the number of calories you burn per day. Some of that comes from the energy your cells use to perform everyday lifesaving functions (like maintaining heart muscle contractions that keep your blood flowing). That's called your *basal metabolic rate.* You also burn calories through activity, whether that's taking out the garbage or running a 5-K. The last piece of the metabolism puzzle comes from digesting your food, which burns calories. This is called the *thermic effect* of food. The sum of all the calories you burn (basal + activity + digestion) equals your total metabolism or total metabolic rate.

Being less active affects your metabolism in two ways: It makes the second "plus" in this equation smaller, but you also lose muscle, which reduces the basal number in the equation.

vitamins and minerals. Carbohydrates, protein, and fat get broken down even further into sugars, amino acids, and fatty acids, respectively. The sugars go to fuel brain and muscle activity (not to mention the doings of every cell in your body), the amino acids get used to build muscle and bone, and the fats get stored for future energy needs or get used to manufacture hormones and other essential compounds.

Ultimately, hundreds of biochemical reactions occur, and the chemical end products of that burger have thousands of uses. But you can see that the ultimate job of your digestive system is to extract as much nutrition as possible out of everything you put in your mouth. The whole process starts with saliva. Saliva contains digestive enzymes that help break the chemical bonds holding foods together so they can be easily crushed and macerated by your teeth. These enzymes are pretty fast acting; if you put a cracker or piece of toast on your tongue, you'll notice it quickly breaking down, even before you start to chew. Your tongue helps position the food in your mouth and moves it to the back of your throat toward your esophagus, the 10-inch connector between your mouth and your stomach. It's different from your windpipe, or trachea, which connects your mouth to your lungs. When you swallow, a little flap called the epiglottis covers the opening of the trachea to guard against choking. (If you've ever had food "go down the wrong way," it's because your epiglottis didn't cover your trachea quickly enough.)

Once in the esophagus, rhythmic automatic muscle contractions help push the food toward your stomach. There, acids further break down your meal, while your stomach muscles churn the whole mixture into what amounts to a nutrient-dense purée, which is then pushed into the 22-foot-long tunnel that is your small intestine. There, with the help of bile, a fat emulsifier produced by your gall bladder, and additional enzymes produced by your pancreas, your meal is absorbed through the walls of your intestine into your bloodstream in the form of individual nutrient building blocks—sugars, fatty acids, and amino acids from carbohydrates, fats, and proteins, respectively. Vitamins and minerals are also absorbed during the journey through the small intestine.

You may have noticed that I didn't mention dietary fiber. That's because you don't absorb fiber. Fiber fills you up, but doesn't add to your overall calorie intake. While fiber does contain as many calories as any other form of carbohydrate—about 4 per gram—your body isn't able to use them for energy. Instead, fiber just moves through your body nearly intact. Along the way, it binds to cholesterol, helping to shuttle it out of your system. A few studies have found that fiber can also prevent absorption of other calories you consume—up to 90 per day.

All the nutrients that enter the bloodstream travel straight to the liver, which filters out wastes and decides where everything usable should go. Anything that isn't absorbed—fiber and waste by-products—travels down into the large intestine and finally through the colon and rectum. Before it leaves your body, small amounts of water and minerals are absorbed in a last-ditch effort to extract every last drop of importance out of that turkey sandwich. Now that you're familiar with your GI tract, let's take a closer look at what's going on when you feel like a beach ball has taken up residence there.

Gas, Solids, and Liquids: The Balloon Gang

THINK OF ONE OF THOSE very long, narrow balloons that you find at a child's birthday party, the ones that clowns twist into different shapes. That balloon represents your GI tract. Now picture the balloon filled with water, air, or solid food. Each of these substances expands the balloon but does so in a different way.

 GAS When air enters the intestine—say, for example, from chewing gum, talking, drinking fizzy drinks, or even smoking—it doesn't get absorbed into the bloodstream. Instead, this gas remains trapped until it can be eventually expelled via a belch or flatulence. Until then, it meanders through your GI tract, causing distension and discomfort.

 SOLID It's generally just a matter of time before solid food gets broken down and absorbed or expelled. But until then, you're feeling like a beached whale.

 LIQUID Just like solid foods, liquid eventually gets absorbed, but sometimes we retain more fluid than our body really needs, resulting in uncomfortable swelling and bloating. Some causes include lifestyle choices such as a nutrient-deficient diet, lack of exercise, and excessive alcohol consumption, while other causes are drug-related or the result of a particular medical problem.

Making Weight

THE FOUR-DAY FLAT ABS KICKSTART eliminates the foods, beverages, and behaviors in your life that cause you to feel uncomfortably full and your stomach to expand. Using the same secret used by elite athletes (such as wrestlers and boxers) who need to make weight to fight in a certain weight class, you'll be doing away with water retention to jumpstart your weight loss. Losing water is not the same as burning fat (we'll tackle that in the next chapter!), but it still creates a major change in your appearance and confidence level. That's not to say you won't lose some serious weight!

Did You Know

A half gallon of water weighs 4 pounds, but if you drink a half gallon of water, you won't gain 4 pounds of fat.

You will, however, temporarily weigh 4 pounds more on the scale—that is, until your kidneys eliminate that water. That's because when you step on that scale, you are weighing anything that has weight to it—the water you just drank, the undigested food you ate a few hours ago, the waste from the food you ate yesterday that hasn't worked its way through your GI tract yet, your muscle mass, skeleton, body fat, and the clothes you're wearing (if any).

Most of the weight fluctuations we see on a scale have to do with our fluid status, because that's the variable that changes the most from hour to hour and day to day. If you're retaining water, you could easily weigh 5 pounds more, and if you're dehydrated (maybe from being sick), you could weigh 5 pounds less. Changes in actual body fat, however, happen much slower and are controlled solely by calories. It takes an excess of 3,500 calories (that means above and beyond the calories you burn) to create 1 pound of body fat. If you ate 700 calories more than your body could burn in a day, you'd gain $1/_5$ of a pound. Do that 5 days in a row starting on a Monday, and by the end of the workweek, you've accumulated 1 pound of fat. (By the way, a pound of fat is nothing to sneeze at; it's equal to four sticks of butter!) So, while that number staring back at you seems to jump up and down like a yo-yo, you can see that it really takes several days in a row of overeating to even gain 1 pound of body fat. The scale is much less fickle when it comes to fat than water!

If you follow the instructions provided for the next 4 days, we estimate that you can expect to lose as much as 4 pounds and up to 3 inches from your waist, hips, thighs, chest, and arms combined. I didn't make these numbers up. They are actual amounts lost, all calculated by an expert who weighed and measured our test panelists. Rest assured: This plan has been proven to work on real men just like you.

While exercise is optional, we strongly recommend that you take a quick 5-minute walk after every meal because moving your body will help your digestive system work at an optimum level. And keep in mind that lifting weights or engaging in any other type of exercise will speed your weight loss and improve your results. So if you are already going to the gym on a regular basis, by all means, keep up the good work! Pro athletes looking to make weight use physical activity to help them drop pounds, and, if possible, so should you.

Four Days: What to Avoid

■ **THE SALT SHAKER, SALT-BASED SEASONINGS, AND HIGHLY PRO-CESSED FOODS:** Water is attracted to sodium, so when you take in higher than usual amounts of sodium, you'll temporarily retain more fluid—which contributes to a sluggish feeling and extra water weight. Cutting back on sodium and boosting your water intake will help bring your body back into balance. It'll also help reduce your risks of hypertension (high blood pressure) and osteoporosis. If you find your food lacks flavor without a few shakes of salt, use the recommended salt-free seasonings.

■ **EXCESS CARBS:** As a backup energy source, your muscles store a type of carbohydrate called glycogen. Every gram of glycogen is stored with about 3 grams of water. But unless you're running a marathon tomorrow, you don't need all this stockpiled fuel. Decrease your intake of high-carbohydrate foods such as pasta, bananas, bagels, and pretzels to temporarily train your body to access this stored fuel and burn it off. At the same time, you'll be getting rid of all that excess stored fluid.

BULKY RAW FOODS: A half-cup serving of cooked carrots delivers the same nutrition as 1 cup raw, but it takes up less room in your GI tract. Eat only cooked vegetables, smaller portions of unsweetened dried fruit, and canned fruits in natural juice. This will allow you to meet your nutrient needs without expanding your GI tract with extra volume.

GASSY FOODS: Certain foods simply create more wind in your GI tract. They include beans and pulses, cauliflower, broccoli, Brussels sprouts, cabbage, onions, peppers, and citrus fruits.

CHEWING GUM: You probably don't realize this, but when you chew gum, you swallow air. All that air gets trapped in your GI tract and causes pressure, bloating, and belly expansion.

SUGAR ALCOHOLS: These sugar substitutes, which go by the names xylitol or maltitol, are often found in low-calorie or low-carb products like biscuits, sweets, and energy bars because they taste sweet. Like fiber, your GI tract can't absorb most of them. That's good for your calorie bottom line but not so good for your belly. Sugar alcohols cause wind, abdominal distention, bloating, and diarrhea. Avoid them.

FRIED FOODS: Fatty foods, especially the fried variety, are digested more slowly, causing you to feel heavy and bloated.

SPICY FOODS: Foods seasoned with black pepper, nutmeg, cloves, chili powder, hot sauces, onions, garlic, mustard, fresh chilies, barbecue sauce, horseradish, ketchup, tomato sauce, or vinegar can all stimulate the release of stomach acid, which can cause irritation.

CARBONATED DRINKS: Where do you think all those bubbles end up? They gang up in your stomach!

ALCOHOL, COFFEE, TEA, HOT COCOA, AND ACIDIC ORANGE JUICE: Each of these high-acid beverages can irritate your GI tract, causing swelling. Herbal tea, which is not made from the leaves of the tea plant, is usually not acidic and is therefore okay to drink during the Kickstart.

Four Days: What to Do

■ **FOLLOW THE FOUR-DAY PLAN EXACTLY.** This includes four 400-calorie meals. This reduces the amount of food in your digestive system at any one time, cuts back on the release of stomach acids, and gets your body used to a regular meal schedule, which you'll continue to follow on the rest of the Flat Belly Diet for Men plan.

■ **EAT FOUR MEALS A DAY.** The Kickstart includes fewer calories—about 1,600 daily—than you'll be eating on the Four-Week MUFA Meal Plan, which allows about 2,000 per day. Eating less for these 4 days reduces the amount of food in your GI tract at any one time, cuts back on the release of stomach acids, and gets your body used to a four-meal-a-day schedule.

■ **TAKE A QUICK 5-MINUTE AFTER-MEAL WALK.** Moving your body helps release air that has been trapped in your GI tract, relieving pressure and bloating. All it takes is a leisurely stroll down your street, around your office building, or around the shops or a quick walk with your dog or your family after dinner—anything that gets you moving for just 5 minutes. You can walk for longer if you like, but go at least 5 minutes to get things moving inside your belly. And, as we mentioned above, there's no good reason not to engage in additional exercise (lifting weights, playing tennis, going for a run, whatever), since doing so will only improve your results and increase you metabolism.

■ **DRINK ONE 2-LITER SERVING OF FIRE WATER EVERY DAY.** A hallmark of this plan is Milton's specialty water, which we've dubbed Fire Water, flavored with fresh ingredients. You'll find the recipe below. We call it Fire Water because it has a bit more of a kick than plain old water. But the ingredients aren't just for flavor: The ginger and mint help calm and soothe your

GI tract, and cayenne may boost metabolism. Even more important: The simple act of making this Fire Water every day will serve as a reminder for these 4 days that life is a little bit different, that things are going to change. It will keep you focused on the weight loss task ahead.

Fire Water

THE NIGHT BEFORE, fill two 1-liter sports bottles with water, squeeze some lime juice into the water, then add the remaining lime and all other ingredients. Shake vigorously. Allow flavors to meld overnight. Drink 2 liters daily during the 4 days of the Kickstart.

Eat slowly. Often, when you eat quickly, you take in large gulps of air without realizing it. All that excess air gets trapped in your digestive system and causes bloating (think of a balloon stretched to capacity). Taking your time will help prevent the expansion. It will also keep you calm as you eat. Too often, we hurry through meals, always trying to get to the next block of time on our schedule. Let's put an end to this for these 4 days and beyond and remember the joy that comes from respecting mealtimes.

Fire Water

½ teaspoon grated fresh ginger

1 small cucumber, peeled and thinly sliced

1 lime, quartered, seeds removed

6 mint leaves

3–4 dashes hot sauce (such as Frank's RedHot or Tabasco)

Note: If you're really pressed for time, use powdered ginger instead of fresh. It won't be as effective in soothing your stomach, but it's better than nothing. You can also skip peeling the cucumber, though the peel may add a slightly bitter taste.

Track Your Progress

DID YOU KNOW THAT PEOPLE who write down what they eat and when they exercise get much better results than people who don't write anything down? A study of 1,700 overweight and obese Americans showed that participants who kept a log of what they ate lost *twice as much* weight as the participants who

YOU ASK, WE ANSWER

BEFORE YOU GET STARTED, here are some of the questions our test panelists asked. Knowing the answers ahead of time will give you an edge to extra weight loss by helping you achieve even better results!

 What if I don't like some of the meals in the meal plan? During the Four-Day Kickstart, we've asked you to stick to the set menu, which is carefully designed to give you balanced nutrition in the optimal amount of 1,600 calories daily. This will help you get used to cooking and eating the Flat Belly Diet for Men way.

 Is it important for me to measure my food? Yes. For accuracy, we request that you measure all of your food in the Kickstart—especially those that pack a lot of calories in small amounts, including oil, nuts, seeds, peanut butter, avocado, pasta, rice, and oatmeal. Measuring will help ensure that this carefully calculated plan gives you the results you're looking for. Without measuring, it's very easy to accumulate extra calories. Milton has certainly seen this in his practice as a registered dietitian. For cup and spoon measurements ($\frac{1}{2}$ cup, 1 tablespoon, etc.), be sure to level the top. It only takes an extra minute to measure food for the whole meal. And let's be honest, do you know anyone who can accurately free pour 1 tablespoon of oil?

What if I'm allergic to something on the plan? For the Kickstart, you should stick as closely to the plan as possible. If you have an allergy, however, do not hesitate to swap a similar ingredient. If you are allergic to eggs, for example, you can increase the protein portion to have double meat. You may need to repeat a previous meal or specific ingredient that you are not allergic to.

Are there certain beverages I can and cannot drink? During the Four-Day Kickstart, it's best to stick with plain water or herbal tea. Or, of course, Fire Water. If possible, please limit coffee and alcohol consumption because both add extra calories to the diet. (Black coffee and unsweetened caffeinated tea don't add calories but can irritate your digestion; and of course, any milk or sugar adds calories.)

 What if I don't like Fire Water? Skip the hot sauce. Or, just opt for plain water instead.

didn't write anything down![1] Studies have also shown that people who track their exercise lose more weight than people who don't.[2]

For the Four-Day Flat Abs Kickstart, I've given you a little space on the next few pages to record your observations. It may be helpful to track how your mood changes before and after you eat or exercise or to note when you find it most challenging to stay on the plan. Also, for each meal, assess your hunger or fullness status using the following scale:

1 = STARVING. You may feel shaky, about to pass out, or want to devour the first thing you see and have a hard time slowing down.

3 = MILD TO MODERATE HUNGER. You have physical symptoms of hunger like a growling tummy and that "I need to eat soon" feeling, but you aren't starving or experiencing any unpleasant symptoms such as a headache, shaking, etc.

5 = JUST RIGHT. Your hunger is gone. You feel satisfied and full but not too full. Your mind is off food, and you're ready to take on the next task. You feel energized.

8 = OVERLY FULL. You think you overdid it. Your tummy feels stretched and uncomfortable. You may feel kind of sluggish, not energized at all.

10 = STUFFED! As in, the way you feel after a huge Thanksgiving dinner.

The Lowdown on Gas

Gas and bloating is a common condition, but in some cases, it can be a sign of a more serious health problem. It's time to see a doctor when

You're suffering from chronic constipation, diarrhea, nausea, or vomiting.

You have persistent abdominal or rectal pain or heartburn.

You've lost weight without trying.

You have a fever you can't explain.

There is blood in your urine.

Check in with yourself before, during, and after you eat. Aim to eat when your hunger is at 3. Stop eating when your fullness and satisfaction level has reached about 5.

Day 4 and Beyond

As you reach the final day of your Flat Abs Kickstart, I know you'll be feeling stronger and healthier than you've felt in a long time. And that's exactly the right mindset for moving ahead and beginning the next phase of the Flat Belly Diet for Men: the Four-Week MUFA Meal Plan that will give you the tools to lose weight, build muscle, and flatten your abs, once and for all.

Four-Day Flat Abs Kickstart Shopping List

PRODUCE

- ❑ Apples, any variety, 2 medium
- ❑ Avocado (Florida), 1 ripe
- ❑ Baby carrots, 10-ounce bag
- ❑ Banana, 1 medium
- ❑ Cherry tomatoes, 1 pint fresh
- ❑ Cremini mushrooms, 1 cup
- ❑ Cucumbers, 4 medium
- ❑ Ginger (2" piece), fresh
- ❑ Grapes, seedless, 1 bunch
- ❑ Green beans, 8 ounces fresh or 9 ounces frozen
- ❑ Lettuce (for sandwiches), head or small bag
- ❑ Limes, 4 medium
- ❑ Melon, any variety, 1 cup fresh or frozen
- ❑ Mint, 2 bunches fresh
- ❑ Sweet potato, 2 (5" each)
- ❑ Tomato, 1 large
- ❑ Yellow peppers, 2–3 large

GROCERY/ REFRIGERATED

- ❑ Sabra Roasted Red Pepper Hummus, 10-ounce container

DAIRY

- ❑ Cheddar cheese, low-fat slices, 6-ounce package
- ❑ Eggs, 2 large
- ❑ Laughing Cow Mini Babybel Original Semisoft Cheese, 2 packages (6 per package)
- ❑ Milk, fat-free, 1 gallon
- ❑ Plain Greek Yogurt, Stonyfield Farm Oikos Organic, 2 cups
- ❑ Vanilla Ice Cream, Breyers Natural, 1.5 quart (or smaller if available in market)

MEAT/SEAFOOD

- ❑ Chicken breast, 4 ounces uncooked
- ❑ Cod fillet, 6 ounces uncooked
- ❑ Deli ham, all-natural low-sodium smoked uncured, 4 ounces
- ❑ Deli roast beef, all-natural low-sodium top round, 6 ounces
- ❑ Ground turkey breast, 93% lean, 1 pound (Note: You will not use all the turkey on the Kickstart; you may want to freeze the rest to use during the Four-Week MUFA Meal Plan.)
- ❑ Pork tenderloin, 4 ounces uncooked

DRY GOODS

- ❑ Almonds, smoked/roasted/raw, 9-ounce jar
- ❑ Brown rice, 14-ounce box
- ❑ Cashews, 9-ounce jar
- ❑ Cornflakes, 12-ounce box
- ❑ Cream of Wheat cereal, instant, 12-ounce box
- ❑ English muffins, plain, 6-pack
- ❑ Extra-virgin olive oil, 8-ounce bottle
- ❑ Hot sauce (such as Frank's RedHot or Tabasco), 12-ounce jar
- ❑ Italian dressing, 8-ounce bottle
- ❑ Mayonnaise, 8-ounce jar
- ❑ Pasta, any noodle variety, 16-ounce box
- ❑ Pasta sauce, any variety, 14-ounce jar
- ❑ Raisins, 6 (1-ounce) boxes
- ❑ Ranch dressing, 8-ounce bottle
- ❑ Tahini, 16-ounce jar (or smaller if available in market)
- ❑ Tuna, packed in water, 2 (5-ounce) cans
- ❑ Whole grain bread, 1 loaf (Note: You will not use all the bread on the Kickstart; you may want to freeze the rest to use during the Four-Week MUFA Meal Plan.)
- ❑ Whole wheat pita, 12-ounce pack (6 pita breads) (Note: You will not use all the pita bread on the Kickstart; you may want to freeze the rest to use during the Four-Week MUFA Meal Plan.)

DRY SPICES (OPTIONAL)

- ❑ Basil
- ❑ Bay leaf
- ❑ Cardamom powder
- ❑ Cinnamon
- ❑ Curry powder
- ❑ Dill
- ❑ Ginger
- ❑ Marjoram
- ❑ Oregano
- ❑ Paprika
- ❑ Rosemary
- ❑ Sage
- ❑ Tarragon
- ❑ Thyme
- ❑ Turmeric

THE FOUR-DAY FLAT ABS KICKSTART, DAY 1

BREAKFAST

- ☐ 2 cups unsweetened cornflakes
- ☐ 1 ½ cups fat-free milk
- ☐ 1 medium apple, peeled

CALORIES: 397

Hunger before:

Hunger after:

Observations:

LUNCH

- ☐ 2 ounces all-natural low-salt smoked uncured ham
- ☐ 2 slices whole grain bread
- ☐ Lettuce & tomato, sliced
- ☐ 2 teaspoons mayonnaise
- ☐ 1 cup raw sweet yellow pepper
- ☐ 1 tablespoon ranch dressing

Assemble the ham, lettuce, and tomato on the bread with mayonnaise as a sandwich. Dip the yellow pepper into the ranch dressing as a side.

CALORIES: 400

Hunger before:

Hunger after:

Observations:

Hunger Rating

1 = Starving
You may feel shaky, about to pass out, or want to devour the first thing you see and have a hard time slowing down.

3 = Mild to moderate hunger
You have physical symptoms of hunger like a growling tummy, but you aren't starving or shaky yet.

DATE: _____

SNACK

☐ 3 tablespoons cashews

☐ Banana

☐ Stonyfield Farm Oikos Organic Greek
    Yogurt (Plain)

CALORIES: 369

Hunger before:

Hunger after:

Observations:

DINNER

☐ 1 cup cooked brown rice

☐ 4 ounces raw skinless chicken breast

☐ 1 tablespoon olive oil

☐ 1 cup cooked green beans

Cook brown rice according to package
directions. Meanwhile, cut chicken into
strips. Heat the oil in a skillet and add
chicken. Sauté the chicken until no
longer pink. Add desired seasonings.
Either steam fresh green beans or
microwave frozen green beans. Serve
the chicken with rice and green beans.

CALORIES: 408

Hunger before:

Hunger after:

Observations:

5 = Just right	8 = Overly full	10 = Stuffed!
Your hunger is gone. You feel satisfied but not too full. Your mind is off food, and you're ready to take on the next task.	You think you overdid it. Your tummy feels stretched and uncomfortable. You may feel kind of sluggish, not energized at all.	As in, the way you feel after a huge Thanksgiving dinner.

THE FOUR-DAY FLAT ABS KICKSTART, DAY 2

BREAKFAST

- ❑ 2 packets/cups instant Cream of Wheat cereal
- ❑ 1 cup fat-free milk
- ❑ 30 raisins (1 miniature box)

CALORIES: 423

Hunger before:

Hunger after:

Observations:

LUNCH

- ❑ 6 ounces all-natural top round roast beef
- ❑ 1 cup cherry tomatoes
- ❑ 2 tablespoons Italian dressing, drizzled on cherry tomatoes
- ❑ 10 seedless grapes

CALORIES: 396

Hunger before:

Hunger after:

Observations:

SNACK

- ❑ 3 pieces Laughing Cow Mini Babybel Original Semisoft Cheese
- ❑ 4 tablespoons cashews

CALORIES: 410

Hunger before:

Hunger after:

Observations:

Hunger Rating

1 = Starving
You may feel shaky, about to pass out, or want to devour the first thing you see and have a hard time slowing down.

3 = Mild to moderate hunger
You have physical symptoms of hunger like a growling tummy, but you aren't starving or shaky yet.

DATE:

DINNER

- ☐ 6 ounces cod fillet
- ☐ ½ teaspoon extra-virgin olive oil
- ☐ 1 tablespoon fresh lemon juice
- ☐ Black pepper, to taste
- ☐ 1 cup green beans steamed, garlic powder to taste
- ☐ 1 sweet potato (5"), skin removed
- ☐ Cinnamon, pinch
- ☐ 1 teaspoon brown sugar
- ☐ ½ cup Breyers Natural Vanilla Ice Cream

Preheat oven to 350°F. Top fish with olive oil, lemon, and pepper and bake in an ovenproof baking dish for 15 minutes, or until it flakes with a fork. Steam green beans in 2 tablespoons water in a microwave-safe dish for 2 to 3 minutes, or until tender. Sprinkle the cinnamon and brown sugar on the sweet potatoes, and cook in a microwave oven for 7 to 8 minutes. Let stand for 5 minutes; potato will continue to cook. (Microwave cooking times vary depending upon the microwave.) Have the ice cream for dessert.

CALORIES: 410

Hunger before:

Hunger after:

Observations:

5 = Just right	8 = Overly full	10 = Stuffed!
Your hunger is gone. You feel satisfied but not too full. Your mind is off food, and you're ready to take on the next task.	You think you overdid it. Your tummy feels stretched and uncomfortable. You may feel kind of sluggish, not energized at all.	As in, the way you feel after a huge Thanksgiving dinner.

THE FOUR-DAY FLAT ABS KICKSTART, DAY 3

❏ 1 English muffin

❏ 2 eggs

❏ ¼ cup sliced avocado

❏ 1 slice low-fat Cheddar cheese

Poach eggs or fry eggs in a pan coated with cooking spray. Top a toasted English muffin with cooked eggs, avocado slices, and a cheese slice.

CALORIES: 375

Hunger before:

Hunger after:

Observations:

❏ 2 ounces low-salt all-natural smoked uncured ham

❏ Lettuce

❏ Tomato, sliced

❏ 2 slices whole grain bread

❏ 2 teaspoons mayonnaise

❏ 1 cup raw carrots

❏ 1 tablespoon Ranch dressing

Assemble the ham, lettuce, and tomato on the bread with mayonnaise. Dip the carrots into the Ranch dressing as a side.

CALORIES: 410

Hunger before:

Hunger after:

Observations:

Hunger Rating

1 = Starving	3 = Mild to moderate hunger
You may feel shaky, about to pass out, or want to devour the first thing you see and have a hard time slowing down.	You have physical symptoms of hunger like a growling tummy, but you aren't starving or shaky yet.

DATE:

SNACK

- ❏ 1 plain pita
- ❏ 4 tablespoons Sabra Roasted Red Pepper Hummus
- ❏ 1 tablespoon tahini (sesame butter)
- ❏ 1 medium apple, peeled

Fill the pita with hummus and drizzle with the tahini.
Eat the apple on the side.

CALORIES: 403

Hunger before:

Hunger after:

Observations:

DINNER

- ❏ 1 tablespoon olive oil
- ❏ 3 ounces 93% lean ground turkey breast
- ❏ ½ cup cooked pasta
- ❏ ½ cup pasta sauce
- ❏ 1 cup mushrooms, steamed in microwave

Heat the oil in a nonstick skillet and add ground turkey.
Cook until the turkey is no longer pink, or until the internal
temperature is 165°F on a meat thermometer. Cook pasta
according to package directions. Add the cooked
mushrooms to the sauce as desired or serve on the side.
Add the turkey to the pasta and serve with sauce.

CALORIES: 419

Hunger before:

Hunger after:

Observations:

5 = Just right	8 = Overly full	10 = Stuffed!
Your hunger is gone. You feel satisfied but not too full. Your mind is off food, and you're ready to take on the next task.	You think you overdid it. Your tummy feels stretched and uncomfortable. You may feel kind of sluggish, not energized at all.	As in, the way you feel after a huge Thanksgiving dinner.

THE FOUR-DAY FLAT ABS KICKSTART, DAY 4

BREAKFAST:

- ❑ 2 cups unsweetened cornflakes
- ❑ 1½ cups fat-free milk
- ❑ 1 cup melon, fresh or frozen

CALORIES: 380

Hunger before:

Hunger after:

Observations:

LUNCH:

- ❑ 2 (5-ounce) cans chunk light tuna packed in water, drained
- ❑ 2 tablespoons mayonnaise
- ❑ 1 cup sweet yellow pepper strips

Mix drained tuna with mayonnaise and serve with pepper strips on the side.

CALORIES: 395

Hunger before:

Hunger after:

Observations:

Hunger Rating

1 = Starving
You may feel shaky, about to pass out, or want to devour the first thing you see and have a hard time slowing down.

3 = Mild to moderate hunger
You have physical symptoms of hunger like a growling tummy, but you aren't starving or shaky yet.

DATE:

❑ 3 pieces Laughing Cow Mini Babybel Original
    Semisoft Cheese

❑ 2 tablespoons almonds

    CALORIES: 428

Hunger before:

Hunger after:

Observations:

DINNER:

❑ 4 ounces lean pork tenderloin

❑ 1 (4-ounce) sweet potato (5")

❑ 1 tablespoon olive oil

❑ 1 cup cooked green beans

Hunger before:

Hunger after:

Observations:

Preheat oven to 425°F. Roast pork tenderloin sprinkled
with desired seasoning for 15–20 minutes or until the
internal temperature is 160°F on a meat thermometer.
Bake the sweet potato in a microwave oven for 10
minutes or until desired doneness and drizzle with half
the olive oil. Steam or microwave green beans and drizzle
with the remaining olive oil. Serve pork with sweet potato
and green beans on the side.

CALORIES: 428

5 = Just right	8 = Overly full	10 = Stuffed!
Your hunger is gone. You feel satisfied but not too full. Your mind is off food, and you're ready to take on the next task.	You think you overdid it. Your tummy feels stretched and uncomfortable. You may feel kind of sluggish, not energized at all.	As in, the way you feel after a huge Thanksgiving dinner.

READ A FLAT BELLY
SUCCESS
STORY

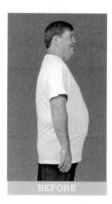

BEFORE

AFTER

Jim
Doherty

AGE: 48

POUNDS LOST:

13.4

IN 32 DAYS

ALL-OVER
INCHES LOST:

6

3.5 FROM
THE WAIST

**↘ favorite
mini meal**
Greek Tortilla
Pizza, *page 125*

"What I learned most of all on the Flat Belly Diet for Men is that I don't have to starve myself to loose weight. The recipes and food in the Flat Belly Diet for Men were filling and simple to make even with a busy schedule," says Jim, a 48-year-old sales rep and deputy fire chief. Jim not only lost 13 pounds on the plan, he also gained the respect of his doctor.

Jim's weight problems began a few years after high school when he stopped playing football and started to pack on the pounds. He gained steadily over the years, and by the time he was 48 years old, he was 70 pounds overweight. Then, 7 years ago, Jim was diagnosed with type 2 diabetes. "I started with oral medications, which helped," says Jim. "But they never brought my blood sugar down within normal ranges, so I began giving myself insulin shots twice a day and increased the dosages of the oral medications."

With his doctor's urging, Jim tried to lose weight, but on other diets he would lose a few pounds only to eventually put the weight back on. However, after losing more than 13 pounds and $3\frac{1}{2}$ inches from his waist on the Flat Belly Diet for Men (and keeping it off), Jim's doctor stopped his daily injections and cut his oral medication by half. And instead of his usual average of 225 mg/dL for fasting blood sugar in the morning,

Jim now gets a reading of 90 to 110—an amount considered ideal. "Besides the diabetes, my blood pressure is better, too. My doctor measured it, and he was thrilled. What a good feeling to let my doctor see this progress."

Eating better and losing weight gave Jim more energy and the stimulation he needed to begin exercising again. Jim's wife, Sharon, reports that she now has trouble keeping pace with him when they go for walks in the park. In fact, Jim joked that he was recently able to lap Sharon for the first time. "Initially I couldn't keep up with my wife, but now it's reversed," he adds.

Jim has learned to make his exercise a priority. "I plan ahead to work it in. Exercise, just like eating right, is now just a regular part of my day. The Flat Belly Diet for Men is not just a 'diet,' it's a way of life."

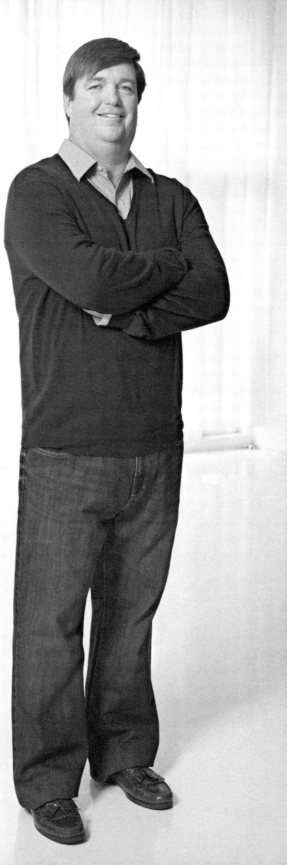

THE FLAT BELLY DIET
FOR MEN
RULES

YOU'VE JUST SUCCESSFULLY finished a major milestone on the Flat Belly Diet for Men—the Four-Day Flat Abs Kickstart! Hopefully, seeing your spare tire deflate over the past 4 days has given you the push needed to move on to the next—and most life-changing—phase of the Flat Belly Diet for Men. Are you ready to lose that gut?

If you've tried other weight loss plans before, the word *diet* probably conjures up a host of negative images: long lists of forbidden foods, feeling tired, being hungry 24/7, gaining all the weight back as soon as you return to normal eating. That's why we created a plan designed to work for all guys, all the time. How did we do it? Milton drew on his years counseling men on weight loss issues to pinpoint the key things guys want in an eating plan.

■ **FOCUS ON HEALTH AND ENERGY.** The Flat Belly Diet for Men will help you get lean, healthy, and strong. You'll drop pounds (not muscle), and you'll gain the energy and stamina you need to perform better at work, on the sports field, in the gym, on the track, and hey, even in bed. Featuring satisfying and energizing foods packed with protein, fiber, and MUFAs, this 2,000-calorie-a-day diet is as healthy and filling as they come.

FLEXIBILITY. If you're pressed for time (who isn't?) or just hate cooking, we wanted you to be able to throw together meals quickly, with little or no cooking. If, on the other hand, you enjoy cooking, you should be able to do so without it impacting your heath goals. The flexibility doesn't stop there. If you don't like a suggested meal, you can swap it out for something you do want to eat. You can eat the same few meals over and over if that's what you prefer. It's that simple.

FLAVOR. Even if you're not a big-time foodie, no diet is complete unless the food is delicious and the meals are palatable. What's the point of being on an eating plan if the food isn't good? This diet offers as much taste as nutrition.

The Three Flat Belly Diet for Men Rules

OVER THE NEXT 28 DAYS—and beyond—you are not only going to lose weight, you're also going to eat very well. As we mentioned above, flavor and flexibility were two key ingredients we made sure to build into your Four-Week MUFA Meal Plan. In Chapter 7, we've given you almost 100 quick-fix meals that are perfect for guys who are too busy to cook or those who just don't like spending time in the kitchen. If cooking is your thing, though, or you want to impress your mate with your culinary skills, Chapter 8 is loaded with mouthwatering MUFA-packed recipes, including a section on grilling that will really get your taste buds going.

Feel free to mix and match any of these meals, in any combination, at any time—provided you stick to three important eating commandments.

You must stick to these rules if you expect to reap the health and weight loss rewards of this plan—and to eliminate that gut. They are:

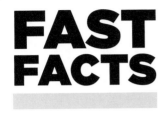

FAST FACTS

One pound of fat is the equivalent of four sticks of butter. Imagine four sticks of butter gone from your abs. This is what you can do for yourself by following the Flat Belly Diet for Men!

RULE #1: Stick to 400 calories per meal.

RULE #2: Never go more than 4 hours without eating.

RULE #3: Eat a MUFA at every meal.

Rule #1: Stick to 400 Calories per Meal

It may have occurred to you at some point while reading this book that MUFA-rich foods aren't exactly low-cal options. Many of these foods—nuts, oils, dark chocolate—are ones that you'd probably avoid on other weight loss programs. But MUFAs are central to this plan because of their ability to reduce belly fat, which makes calorie control more important than ever. All meals and snacks in the Flat Belly Diet for Men include a MUFA and provide about 400 calories. An added bonus of this controlled-calorie plan is that you can substitute one whole meal for another. For example, you can eat breakfast for dinner or lunch for breakfast. Or if you love lunch meals, you can even eat five of them in one day. It really doesn't make a difference. That's the ease of this diet.

The goal for this plan is to have five meals a day, bringing your daily calorie count to 2,000. This is how many calories it takes for a man of average height, frame size, and activity level to get to and stay at his ideal body weight. It's enough calories to keep up your energy, support your immune system, and maintain your necessary calorie-burning muscle. Not only that, the meals in this plan focus on the powerhouse nutrient protein, to keep your energy levels up, and are full of fiber, so you don't get hungry. The result? You won't feel tired, cranky, moody, or famished, but you also won't be eating enough calories to hold on to that spare tire.

Rule #2: Never Go More Than 4 Hours without Eating

Clearly, a diet isn't going to work if you're hungry or tired all the time. That's why you must eat every 4 hours while on the Flat Belly Diet for Men. If you wait too long, you can become so hungry (and cranky) that you stop thinking straight. Once this kicks in, you'll lose the energy and patience to pick the healthiest meal choice, let alone prepare one. You know that feeling, right? The hunger sets in and suddenly you're grabbing anything in sight (a bag of chips, fast food, cookies, you name it) and aren't able to stop eating.

In light of this, snacks are a central part of this diet, and you should eat two a day. However, when you eat these snacks is entirely up to you. Some people prefer to snack post-dinner (we've included some dessert-style snacks for this purpose), while others need a little energy boost in the middle of the afternoon. Your snack time is entirely yours and entirely necessary. To help you include two snacks every day, Milton has created a variety of Power Snacks that you can prepare ahead of time and carry with you. They're portable, easy to assemble, and MUFA-loaded. You can even use these Power Snacks as a floating meal.

Rule #3: Eat a MUFA at Every Meal

"A MUFA at every meal"—just keep repeating that to yourself. As you already know, MUFA stands for monounsaturated fatty acid. These heart-healthy, disease-fighting, "good" fats are found in foods like almonds, peanut butter, olive oil, olives, avocados, and even dark chocolate. MUFAs are an unsaturated fat and have the exact opposite effect of the unhealthy saturated and trans fats

YOUR MUFA SERVING CHART

FOOD	SERVING	CALORIES
SOYBEANS (EDAMAME), SHELLED AND BOILED	1 cup	244
SEMISWEET CHOCOLATE CHIPS	1/4 cup	207
ALMOND BUTTER	2 Tbsp	200
CASHEW BUTTER	2 Tbsp	190
SUNFLOWER SEED BUTTER	2 Tbsp	190
NATURAL PEANUT BUTTER, CRUNCHY	2 Tbsp	188
NATURAL PEANUT BUTTER, SMOOTH	2 Tbsp	188
TAHINI (SESAME SEED PASTE)	2 Tbsp	178
PUMPKIN SEEDS (WITHOUT THE SHELL)	2 Tbsp	148
CANOLA OIL	1 Tbsp	124
FLAXSEED OIL (COLD-PRESSED ORGANIC)	1 Tbsp	120
MACADAMIA NUTS	2 Tbsp	120
SAFFLOWER OIL (HIGH OLEIC)	1 Tbsp	120
SESAME OR SOYBEAN OIL	1 Tbsp	120
SUNFLOWER OIL (HIGH OLEIC)	1 Tbsp	120
WALNUT OIL	1 Tbsp	120
OLIVE OIL	1 Tbsp	119
PEANUT OIL	1 Tbsp	119
PINE NUTS	2 Tbsp	113
BRAZIL NUTS	2 Tbsp	110
HAZELNUTS	2 Tbsp	110
PEANUTS	2 Tbsp	110
ALMONDS	2 Tbsp	109
KALAMATA OLIVES	10 large	105
CASHEWS	2 Tbsp	100
CANOLA OIL MAYONNAISE	1 Tbsp	100
AVOCADO, CALIFORNIA (HASS)	1/4 cup	96
SESAME SEEDS (WITH THE SHELL)	2 Tbsp	91
PECANS	2 Tbsp	90
SUNFLOWER SEEDS (WITHOUT THE SHELL)	2 Tbsp	90
BLACK OLIVE TAPENADE	2 Tbsp	88
PISTACHIOS	2 Tbsp	88
WALNUTS	2 Tbsp	82
PESTO	1 Tbsp	80
AVOCADO, FLORIDA	1/4 cup	69
GREEN OLIVE TAPENADE	2 Tbsp	54
GREEN OR BLACK OLIVES	10 large	50

you might have heard about in the news. Chances are you'll look forward to adding these super fats to your meals because they taste great, whether you drizzle olive oil over your favorite meal or grab a handful of almonds.

You'll find MUFA-rich foods incorporated into every meal and Power Snack in this eating plan. If you don't like certain MUFAs, you can substitute one for another as long as the calorie counts are nearly the same. For example, you can exchange avocado (96 calories) for cashews (100 calories). For precise MUFA serving amounts per meal, consult page 99. Better yet, copy this chart and post it somewhere easily accessible. To get better acquainted with the five MUFA groups and to learn how to buy, store, and prepare them, turn to pages 105–113.

The Nutrition Guidelines

HERE ARE A FEW GENERAL guidelines to keep in mind to help you eat and lose weight the Flat Belly Diet for Men way.

Consume no more than 4 grams of saturated fat per meal.

Saturated fat raises levels of LDL ("bad") cholesterol in your blood and, in turn, increases your risk of cardiovascular disease and stroke. Animal products, like meat and dairy products, are the main sources of saturated fat, but tropical oils—coconut oil and palm (or palm kernel) oil—and cocoa butter are also high in saturated fat. Small amounts of saturated fat are also found in some other plant foods, including MUFA-rich olive oil and nuts, so it's impossible to eliminate the saturated fats altogether. However, you can greatly decrease the amount in your diet by substituting healthier fats, like olive oil and canola oil, for straight saturated fats like butter. In your Four-Week MUFA Meal Plan, we've kept the saturated fat level as low as possible, so you see it is possible to have flavor without saturated fats!

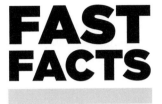

FAST FACTS

With the limit on saturated fats, you might be wondering why dark chocolate is included in the Flat Belly Diet for Men plan. The amount we recommend (¼ cup of semisweet chocolate chips or the equivalent) contains quite a bit more than 3 grams of saturated fat. There are different types of saturated fat, and the type in dark chocolate (stearic acid) largely gets converted in the body to oleic acid, which is a MUFA! So although dark chocolate has a higher saturated fat content—and when you include it in one of your Flat Belly Diet for Men meals, your total saturated fat will be over the 4-gram max—this type does not tend to raise blood cholesterol levels and is considered heart healthy.

Ban trans fat.

Like saturated fat, trans fat increases levels of LDL ("bad") cholesterol in your blood. But that's not all. Trans fat also lowers levels of HDL ("good") cholesterol, which helps keep blood vessels clear, making trans fat a really bad fat. Trans fat is produced when hydrogen is added to liquid oils to make them solid (and extend their shelf life), and it is found mostly in packaged products. Because manufacturers are allowed to claim zero trans fat for any food containing up to half a gram per serving, it's important to identify trans fats in the ingredients list. Look for the words hydrogenated, partially hydrogenated, and shortening. If you spot these terms in the list, put that food down and keep looking!

Avoid artificial sweeteners, flavorings, and preservatives.

Artificial sweeteners, like aspartame, sucralose, and saccharin, are commonly found in diet sodas, sugar-free yogurts and puddings, chewable vitamins, gum, and even high-fiber cereal. Aspartame is one of the most prevalent, but ever since the FDA approved it in 1981, many nutrition researchers have disputed its safety, and many people have complained that it causes headaches, dizziness, and mood changes. Artificial food colorings used in some sugary cereals and candies have been linked to hyperactivity and behavior problems since the 1970s. Nitrates, which add flavor (mostly to meats), have been linked to various types of cancer. And these are just a few of the many artificial additives in our food. Try to avoid artificial anything (colors, flavors, preservatives). Instead, pick whole foods as often as possible and look for foods with ingredients you can easily recognize and pronounce.

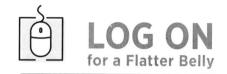

LOG ON
for a Flatter Belly

Check out **www.prevention.com**, where you can find:
- More delicious MUFA-packed, calorie-controlled Flat Belly Diet recipes
- Personal health trackers where you can record what you eat, how much you exercise, and other customizable health measurements
- Success stories from women and men of all shapes and sizes who have lost weight with the Flat Belly Diet

Limit sodium to less than 2,300 milligrams a day.

Sodium causes water retention and increases your risk for high blood pressure, which can lead to heart and kidney disease, as well as stroke. Because the Flat Belly Diet for Men is about flattening your belly and enhancing good health, it recommends keeping your total sodium below 2,300 milligrams a day (or approximately 575 milligrams per meal).

YOU ASK, WE ANSWER

BEFORE YOU GET STARTED, here are some of the questions our test panelists asked. Knowing the answers ahead of time will give you an edge to extra weight loss by helping you achieve even better results!

Q Can I eat the same meals every day? If you find a few favorite meals you really like, by all means feel free to repeat them as many times as you like. For the best balance in nutrition, though (and to stave off boredom), we encourage you to choose meals with different MUFAs each day. This is especially important with dark chocolate, which is a little higher in sugar than other MUFAs, and with olives, which are a little higher in sodium than other MUFAs.

Q Do I have to stick to meals from the book? For the duration of the Four-Week MUFA Meal Plan, it's probably best to stick with meals and recipes you'll find in this book, which have been carefully designed to give you a good balance of protein, carbs, and MUFAs—not to mention taste! Once you've become accustomed to eating 400-calorie meals with a MUFA, we encourage you to experiment a little to make your own MUFA recipes. Just be sure to keep the Flat Belly nutrition guidelines in mind when you do so.

Q Do I still need to measure my food? I know, I know, it gets tiresome to pull out the measuring cups and spoons for every meal. But, as we mentioned in the Kickstart, it's very easy to overdo it if you don't. So for best results, we recommend that you continue to measure your food throughout the Four-Week MUFA Meal Plan. Remember, for cup and spoon measurements ($\frac{1}{2}$ cup, 1 tablespoon, etc.), be sure to level the top.

Q When can I have coffee, beer, and sodas again? You'll lose weight and inches faster if you stick with the calorie- and carbonation-free choices you've been drinking on the Kickstart: plain water, Fire Water, and herbal tea. During the Four-Week MUFA Meal Plan, if you want to add some other beverages for variety, feel free to do so. Black coffee and caffeinated tea (black, green, red, or white) are calorie-free! Just be careful to account for the added calories from milk and sugar. Similarly, make sure you note the calories in any sodas, juices, beer, or other drinks you enjoy. (See page 59 for more on alcohol consumption.)

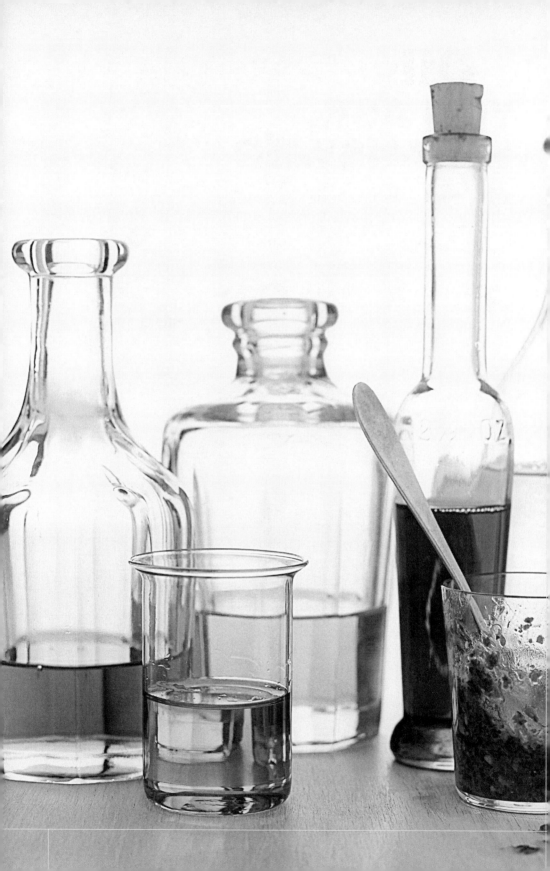

1. Oils

THE MOST VERSATILE MUFA of all, oil is a welcome addition to any meal. Choose your oil based on use (cooking or drizzling) and flavor (strong or mild).

HOW TO BUY AND USE: We recommend going with expeller-pressed oils, a chemical-free extraction process. This natural method allows the oil to retain its natural color, aroma, and nutrients. Cold-pressed oil is expeller pressed in a heat-controlled environment to keep temperatures below 120°F. This is important for delicate oils like flaxseed.

HOW TO STORE: Choose a storage container that holds only what you'll use within 2 months. As each container empties, it fills with oxygen, which causes the oil to oxidize (a fancy way to say deteriorate). This will eventually create a stale or bitter taste (like wet cardboard) and contribute to a breakdown of vitamin E and those precious MUFAs. Opt for dark glass jars or tins (rather than clear plastic bottles) to protect the oil from light, another source of flavor-sapping oxidation. You can store opened bottles of olive, canola, and peanut oils in a dark, cool place, such as the back of your pantry. Flaxseed oil, on the other hand, should always be kept in the refrigerator because it breaks down more quickly at warmer temperatures.

HISTORY: Oils extracted from plant foods have been used in nearly every culture around the globe since ancient times. A 4,000-year-old kitchen unearthed by an archeologist in Indiana revealed that large slabs of rock had been used to crush nuts and then extract the oil.

INSIDE SCOOP!

SAFFLOWER OIL LABELED "HIGH-OLEIC" CONTAINS THE MOST BENEFICIAL MUFAS, FOLLOWED BY OLIVE OIL AND THEN CANOLA OIL.

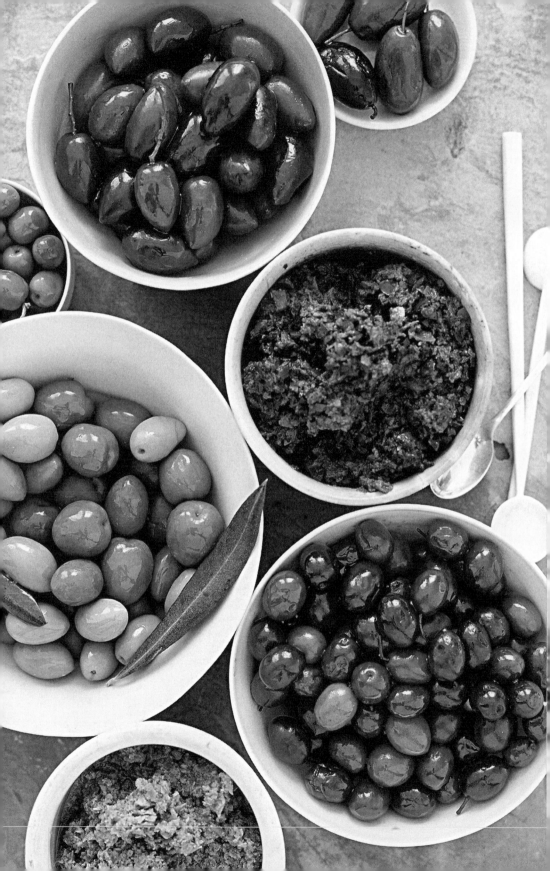

2. Olives

WITH SO MANY CHOICES out there, you're bound to find an olive to your liking. Choose your color (black or green) and pick your flavor (salty, sweet, or spicy). To mix it up, you can switch to tapenade, a delicious spread made from the crushed fruit.

HOW TO BUY AND USE: Fresh olives are available during the summer in specialty markets, but don't take a chance on them unless you're a serious gourmet. Why? They're incredibly bitter and inedible, thanks to a naturally occurring compound called oleuropein. Instead, choose the more appetizing olives at deli counters, which are sometimes pasteurized and cured in oil, salt, or brine, and flavored with herbs or hot chilies. Olives can be purchased in jars and cans, as well as in bulk.

HOW TO STORE: Olives should be stored in the refrigerator after opening, either in a jar or an airtight container. If you bought canned olives, transfer any leftover ones into another airtight container before storing them in the fridge.

HISTORY: Native to coastal regions of the Mediterranean, Asia, and areas of Africa, olives have been cultivated since 6000 BC and are one of the oldest known foods. These MUFAs were brought to America by Spanish and Portuguese explorers during the 15th and 16th centuries and to California missions in the late 18th century. Today, most commercial olives are grown in Spain, Italy, Greece, and Turkey.

INSIDE SCOOP!

ALL TYPES OF OLIVES—KALAMATA, NIÇOISE, PICHOLINE, MANZANILLA, AND MORE—ARE A CONCENTRATED SOURCE OF BELLY-FLATTENING MUFAS.

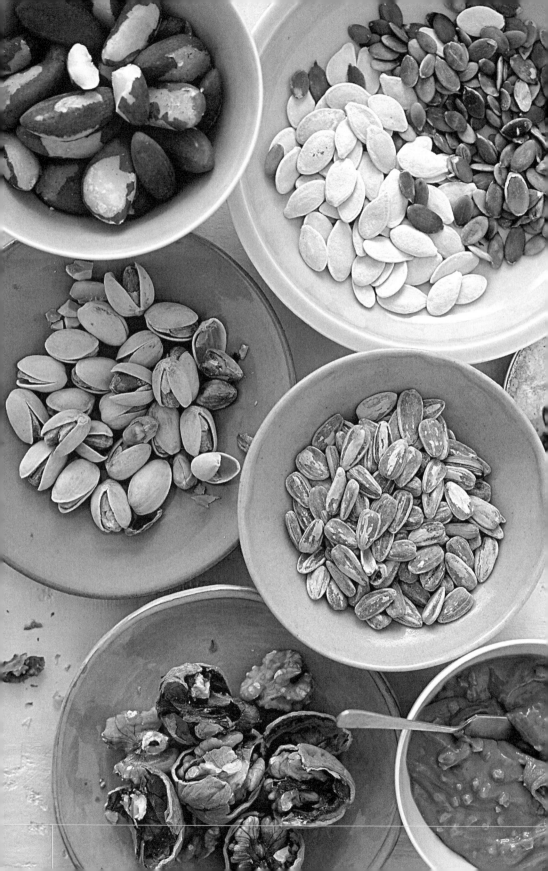

3. Nuts and Seeds

THESE MUFAS HAVE LONG BEEN POPULAR on the health front, thanks to their high levels of protein, fiber, and antioxidants (not to mention those healthy fats). The best part is you can add them to anything really: Sprinkle some on yogurt, cereal, and salads; use them as a topping for fish and chicken; or just snack on them.

HOW TO BUY AND USE: Nuts and seeds are sold in many ways, including vacuum-sealed cans, glass jars, sealed bags, and in bulk. They can be whole, sliced, or chopped; raw or roasted; or in or out of the shell. If purchasing them in bulk, select a market that has a high turnover and uses covered bins to guarantee freshness. Unshelled nuts should be free from cracks or holes, feel somewhat heavy for their size, and should not rattle in the shell. Shelled nuts should be plump and look uniform in size and shape.

HOW TO STORE: Due to their high fat content, nuts and seeds tend to go rancid quickly once their shells are removed, if they're exposed to heat, light, and humidity during storage. When kept in a cool, dry place in an airtight container, raw, unshelled nuts will keep from 6 months to a year, while shelled nuts will stay fresh for 3 to 4 months under the same conditions. Shelled nuts can be stored for 4 months in a refrigerator and 6 months in a freezer.

HISTORY: Nuts and seeds have a long, extensive history. Egypt's pharaohs prized almonds. The use of flaxseed goes as far back as the Stone Age; ancient Greeks and Native Americans have been using sunflower seeds for more than 5,000 years; and peanuts were a staple of the Aztec diet.

INSIDE SCOOP! MACADAMIA NUTS PROVIDE MORE MUFA THAN ANY OTHER NUT OR SEED.

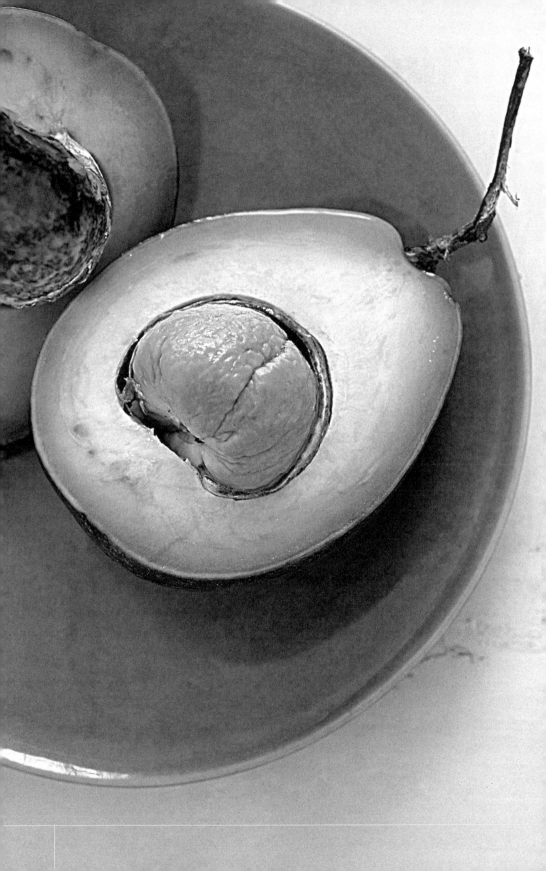

4. **Avocados**

ONCE A LUXURY FOOD reserved for royalty, creamy avocados are now available to the masses. Delicious mashed into a dip or sliced onto a salad, this MUFA is like butter, only much better.

HOW TO BUY AND USE: When selecting an avocado, look for one with slightly soft skin that yields a little when you press it with your thumb. Avoid bruised, cracked, or indented fruit. Those with tear-drop-shaped necks have usually been tree ripened and will have a richer taste than rounded specimens. Once it's ripe, use a sharp knife to slice it lengthwise, guiding the knife gently around the pit. Then twist the two halves against each other in opposite directions to separate. The pit will still be lodged in one half. Carefully nudge the knife into the pit and twist it out to discard. You can either gently peel away the skin or carefully score the avocado while still in the peel, cutting into long slices or chunks. Use a spoon to separate the fruit from the skin.

HOW TO STORE: A whole, ripe avocado with the skin on will keep in the refrigerator for a day or two. A slightly unripe avocado can be ripened in just a day or two by storing it in a paper bag and keeping it on the counter. To prevent a leftover portion from browning, coat the exposed flesh with lemon juice, wrap tightly in plastic wrap, and store in the refrigerator.

HISTORY:

Avocados have been cultivated in South and Central America since 8000 BC. They were not introduced to the United States until the early 20th century, when they were first planted in California and Florida.

INSIDE SCOOP!

HASS AVOCADOS ARE CREAMIER THAN FLORIDA AVOCADOS AND PROVIDE ALMOST TWICE THE MUFA PER ¼-CUP SERVING.

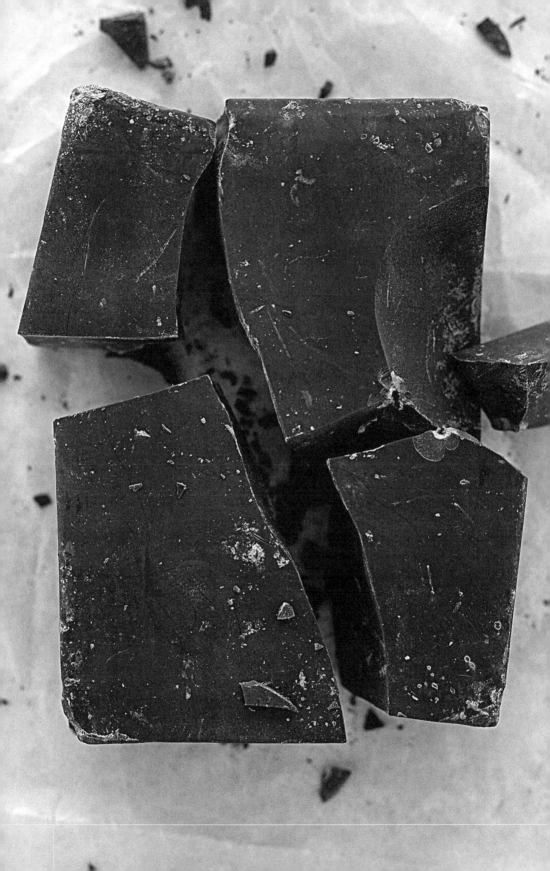

5. Dark Chocolate

YES, IT'S TRUE. You can actually eat chocolate on this eating plan. This beloved MUFA makes every meal or snack a little bit sweeter—and don't deny it, even men love a little (or a lot of) chocolate from time to time.

HOW TO BUY AND USE: Semisweet and other dark chocolates are low enough in sugar and high enough in monounsaturated fats to get the MUFA accolade in our book. Chocolates with a higher cacao, or cocoa, content—the package usually lists the percentage—are typically darker, less sweet, and slightly more bitter, but in a good way. If you're used to milk chocolate, go dark gradually so you train your taste buds to appreciate the stronger flavor of real, dark chocolate. You can buy chocolate in large chunks (popular with the baking set), as molded bars, or in chip form. I like chips because they're so easy to measure and even easier to eat.

HOW TO STORE: Keep dark chocolate that's in its original sealed package in a cool dry area (60°F to 75°F). Once opened, chocolate should be transferred to an airtight container or bag and stashed in the fridge (good) or freezer (best). During prolonged storage, chocolate will often "bloom," or develop a white blush. It's perfectly safe to eat, though not very appetizing to look at. One solution: Melt it and the bloom will disappear.

HISTORY:

You're not the only one who loves chocolate. The ancient Mayans and Aztecs touted it as a food of the gods—and it's been a culinary mainstay ever since.

INSIDE SCOOP!

DARK CHOCOLATE IS RICH IN FLAVONOIDS, WHICH MAY HELP REDUCE BLOOD PRESSURE, PREVENT INFLAMMATION, AND SLOW AGING.

READ A FLAT BELLY
SUCCESS
STORY

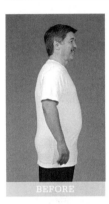
BEFORE

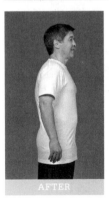
AFTER

Mike Sauer

AGE: 52

POUNDS LOST:

12.8

IN 24 DAYS*

ALL-OVER
INCHES LOST:

11.88

3.5 FROM
THE WAIST

*Due to family circumstances,
Mike was weighed a few days
before the end of the program.

↘ **favorite mini meal**
Yogurt Crunch
Delight, *page 131*

On April 20, 2009, Mike, a 52-year-old fire captain in New Jersey, had a heart attack while on duty at his fire house. "I had responded to several calls during the first part of my 24-hour shift, including a vehicle fire," says Mike. "And at about 5:00 a.m., I woke up with crushing chest pains. At first I thought the pain was related to possible injury or strain from the earlier events, but it wasn't. I was taken to the hospital, where I found out that I had suffered a heart attack. Although the attack was very mild and I have since returned to full duty, my life was changed that day. I was given a second chance and I took advantage of that."

Mike started seeing a nutritionist shortly after the attack, and when she told him about the Flat Belly Diet for Men panel, he immediately signed up. "The Flat Belly Diet for Men helped me turn my health around, and it taught me how to eat . . . the right way."

So, instead of eating just a couple of really large meals each day, Mike follows the set regimen of 400-calorie meals several times a day. And he's come to love the MUFA-packed meals and working out. "I depend on the MUFAs as the core of my diet. They make up every meal or snack. And the exercise maintains my focus and helps me relax. I can think more clearly when it's mealtime, and I can think ahead to figure out my meals for when I'm on duty at the firehouse."

Apparently, losing over 12 pounds is also enough to make a guy stop snoring. "One morning my wife, Terry, announced that I didn't snore last night," says Mike. "I didn't think much of it until she said it again the next morning, and then again the next. This kept happening—or I should say it kept *not* happening. I just stopped snoring. And I don't toss and turn while sleeping. I feel refreshed when I wake up because I sleep much better." While Mike considers it just a nice bonus that he no longer snores, his wife thinks a night's rest without noise is something to celebrate! Another bonus? Losing weight reduced stress on an old knee injury, which has cured his chronic knee pain.

Next up for Mike: joining fellow test panelist Anthony Henry in Las Vegas for a half marathon to benefit the Crohn's & Colitis Foundation of America.

REAL (QUICK)
FLAT BELLY DIET
MEALS
FOR REAL MEN

YOUR FOUR-WEEK MUFA Meal Plan is designed to give you a balanced variety of foods with plenty of MUFA-rich foods to ward off disease, flatten your stomach, and keep you satisfied. But unlike most diets, the Flat Belly Diet for Men doesn't ask you to follow a stringent day-by-day, meal-by-meal menu. Thank goodness! Instead, you'll eat three 400-calorie meals each day, plus two 400-calorie Power Snacks, and *all of the meals are interchangeable.* Meals are categorized here as breakfast, lunch, dinner, and snack, but because every single one follows the Flat Belly "400 calories with a MUFA" rule, you can shuffle them however you like.

There are a number of meals to choose from in each category, so, if you like, you can go for maximum variety and have something different for every meal, every day, for 4 weeks. On the other hand, if you find one lunch you love and want to make it part of your everyday routine, that's fine, too. Bear in mind, though, that it's still important to eat a variety of foods to ensure that you get all the nutrients you need.

Want even more Flat Belly meal options? Turn to Chapter 8, where you'll find more than 50 Flat Belly Diet for Men recipes. You can also check out other books in the *Flat Belly Diet!* series, including the *Flat Belly Diet! Cookbook* and *Flat Belly Diet! Pocket Guide* for additional ideas. Bonus: At the end of this chapter, there's a list of Ready-Made Meals, including meal replacement bars, healthy frozen dinners, and even in-a-pinch fast-food options you can pair with a MUFA serving from the chart on page 99.

The beauty of the Flat Belly Diet for Men is almost nothing is forbidden, so you eat all your favorite foods. But you can't just pair a MUFA with any ol' food or meal and call that a Flat Belly meal. To get the most MUFA for your money, you need to pair them with lean proteins, low-fat dairy, fruits, vegetables, starches, and whole grains. While you might want to start making your own Flat Belly meals right off the bat, it's best to give yourself at least 28 days before you do so. This will give you time to become fully acquainted with the portion sizes, MUFA servings, and basic composition of the meals, and then you will be ready to create your own meals as often as you like. However, customizing the meals to your taste is easy. The two questions on the opposite page will clarify the most important points for you to keep in mind when altering the meals in this chapter.

Meal Numerology

IN THE FOLLOWING MEALS, MUFAs are in boldface, and ingredient calorie counts are in parentheses. These numbers are provided for a few reasons. First, to help you become familiar with the calorie levels of various ingredients—you may be surprised to find out just how many or few calories are in certain foods. The second reason is to help you customize the plan. If you dislike a certain

YOU ASK, WE ANSWER

BEFORE YOU GET STARTED, here are some of the questions our test panelists asked. Knowing the answers ahead of time will give you an edge to extra weight loss by helping you achieve even better results!

Q Do I have to buy these exact brands? Brands have been selected because of their taste, quality, availability, and, most importantly, nutritional value. The nutritional quality of foods in certain categories varies widely, so we scoured the supermarket aisles, read countless labels, and handpicked the high-quality brands that met our tough nutritional standards. Including these foods guarantees steady weight loss because their precise calorie level per serving has been incorporated into the plan. So, yes, I encourage you to use these brands. However, if you can't or prefer not to, simply replace them with comparable foods with as close to the same calorie levels.

Q Can I swap out ingredients in a meal? Yes and no. You should not move items from one meal to another—that is, you can't delete your MUFA from breakfast and add it to lunch. But you *can* swap out foods within a meal, as long as:

■ They're within the same food group, such as tomatoes and red peppers or turkey and chicken; and

■ The food you added provides about the same number of calories as the food you took out. The calories for each ingredient appear in parentheses.

ingredient, don't have the same brand on hand, want to use up something you already have, or want to experiment with a different way of preparing a meal, you can.

Just be sure the food you added provides about the same number of calories as the one you took away. Use the Nutrition Facts label information to check the calorie content of packaged foods; for fresh foods, check out www.prevention.com/healthtracker.

→ Flat Belly Breakfasts

Studies show that breakfast eaters eat less overall and gain less weight than breakfast skimpers. Here, some healthy Flat Belly ways to start your day. MUFAs are in **boldface,** and ingredient calorie counts are in parentheses.

Breakfast Veggie Sandwich:

Crack 2 large eggs (156) into a microwave egg poacher and add ¹⁄₂ cup diced veggies of your choice (16). Cook for 1¹⁄₂ minutes. Top with 1 ounce low-fat Cheddar cheese (48). Layer on 1 toasted whole wheat English muffin (135) spread with 1 tablespoon **pesto** (80).

■ **Total Calories = 435**

Protein Parfait:

Layer ¹⁄₄ cup Bear Naked Peak Protein Original granola (140) with ¹⁄₂ cup Kozy Shack Chocolate Pudding (140), 2 tablespoons **walnuts** (82), and ³⁄₄ cup mandarin oranges, canned in juice (69).

■ **Total Calories = 431**

Pecan Cereal:

Serve 1¹⁄₂ cups Post Original Spoon Size Shredded Wheat cereal (255) with 1 cup fat-free milk (83) and 2 tablespoons **pecans** (90).

■ **Total Calories = 428**

Almond Cereal:

Serve 1 cup Kashi GOLEAN Crunch! cereal (200) with 1 cup fat-free milk (83) and 2 tablespoons slivered **almonds** (109).

■ **Total Calories = 392**

Nutty Breakfast Crunch:

Mix 6 ounces fat-free plain Greek yogurt (60) with ¹⁄₃ cup Grape-Nuts (133) and 2 tablespoons coarsely crushed **macadamia nuts** (120), and top with ¹⁄₂ medium banana, sliced (53).

■ **Total Calories = 366**

Apple Butter Oats:

Cook ¹⁄₂ cup dry Quick Quaker Oats (160) with water to desired consistency. Mix in 3 tablespoons apple butter (87), 2 tablespoons **pecans** (90), and a dash of cinnamon (0). Serve with 1 cup seedless grapes (104).

■ **Total Calories = 441**

Banana Split Oatmeal:

Cook ¹⁄₂ cup dry Quick Quaker Oats (160) with water to desired consistency and mix with ¹⁄₄ cup microwaved frozen strawberries (20). Top with ¹⁄₂ medium banana, sliced (53), 1 tablespoon semisweet chocolate chips (50), and 2 tablespoons **peanuts** (110).

■ **Total Calories = 393**

Nut Butter Burrito:

Spread 2 tablespoons **cashew butter** (190) on 1 Thomas' Sahara 100% Whole Wheat Wrap (170) and top with 1 cup raspberries (64).

■ **Total Calories = 424**

Mediterranean Pita Pocket:

Fill 1 (6¹⁄₂") whole wheat pita (170) with 3 tablespoons hummus (70), 2 tablespoons **tahini** (178), ¹⁄₂ cup shredded romaine lettuce (4),

1/2 cup diced tomato (15), and 1/4 cup diced seedless cucumber (4).

■ **Total Calories = 441**

Bagel Breakfast Sandwich: Toast

1 Thomas' Hearty Grains 100% Whole Wheat Bagel (270) and top with 1 tablespoon part-skim ricotta cheese (21), 2 tablespoons **pine nuts** (113), and 1 ounce lox (33).

■ **Total Calories = 437**

Waffle Sandwich: Toast 2 Van's Origi-

nal Multigrain Waffles (180) and top with 2 tablespoons crunchy **peanut butter** (188) and 2 teaspoons Smucker's Apricot Reduced Sugar Preserves (17).

■ **Total Calories = 385**

Egg Salad Sandwich: Chop 2

large hard-boiled eggs (156) and mix with 1/4 cup diced vegetables, such as tomatoes, celery, or bell peppers (10), a dash of curry powder, and 1 tablespoon Hellman's

canola oil mayonnaise (100). Spread on 2 slices of whole grain bread (160).

■ **Total Calories = 426**

Sunrise Sandwich: Scramble 2 large

eggs in a nonstick pan coated with cooking spray (156). Serve on 2 slices of toasted whole grain bread (160) topped with 1 ounce sliced low-fat baby Swiss cheese (50) and 1/4 cup **Florida avocado** slices (69).

■ **Total Calories = 435**

Breakfast Burrito: Scramble 1/2 cup egg

whites (50) with 2 tablespoons Kraft Natural Mexican Style Four Cheese (50) and 1/4 cup diced vegetables, such as tomatoes, celery, or bell peppers (10). Fill 1 Thomas' Sahara 100% Whole Wheat Wrap (170) with the egg mixture and top with 4 tablespoons Pace Pico de Gallo (20) and 1/4 cup **Hass avocado**, sliced or cubed (96).

■ **Total Calories = 396**

MESSAGE FROM MILTON

Make Breakfast a Flat Belly Must

Clients in my practice often try to save calories and speed weight loss by skipping breakfast. However, what happens again and again is that the "skippers" turn into the losers. Overeating losers, that is. Men who skip their morning meal inevitably compensate by eating more food later in the day. And not just a little more—a *lot* more. If you're not a breakfast person, try something small, like a piece of fruit with a handful of nuts. Or, branch out and try our Flat Belly Sunrise Sandwich (an English muffin with egg and avocado). It's delicious and was the hands-down favorite among our test panelists. It's quick, simple, and tasty.

Grilled Cheese: Spread 1 tablespoon **peanut oil** (119) on one side of each of 2 slices of whole grain bread (160). Make a sandwich with 1.5 ounces provolone cheese (116) and toast in a nonstick skillet.

▪ **Total Calories = 427**

BLT: Toast 2 slices of whole grain bread (160) and top with 1 tablespoon Hellman's **canola oil mayonnaise** (100), 2 slices Niman Ranch Applewood Smoked Bacon (92), 1 slice (1 ounce) Gouda (101), 2 leaves Romaine lettuce, and 3 tomato slices (15).

▪ **Total Calories = 567**

Pizza for Breakfast: Thomas' Sahara Multi-Grain Pita (140) with 2 tablespoons marinara sauce (22), 1 ounce shredded part-skim mozzarella cheese (72), ½ cup diced vegetables of your choice (20), 2 tablespoons **black olive tapenade** (88), and 1 ounce all-natural smoked uncured ham, sliced into thin strips (30). Toast until the cheese melts.

▪ **Total Calories = 372**

Morning Mex Quesadilla: Warm 1 Thomas' Sahara 100% Whole Wheat Wrap (170) in a skillet or microwave oven with ¼ cup Kraft Natural Mexican Style Four Cheese (100) and ¼ cup black beans (50). Add 4 tablespoons Pace Pico de Gallo (20) and 10 large **black olives**, sliced (50). Serve with a clementine (35).

▪ **Total Calories = 415**

→ Flat Belly Lunches

Brown bagging it the Flat Belly way is quick and delish! As with the breakfasts, MUFAs are in **boldface,** and ingredient calorie counts are in parentheses.

Hearty Cobb Salad: Combine 2 cups organic mixed baby greens (18), 3 ounces cooked/roasted chicken breast (122), 1 slice cooked Niman Ranch Applewood Smoked Bacon (46), ½ cup chopped vegetables of your choice (20), 1 medium chopped hard-boiled egg (78), and ¼ cup chopped **Florida avocado** (69). Top with 1 tablespoon Kraft Italian dressing (52).

  ▦ Total Calories = 405

Pesto Chicken Sandwich: Spread 1 Food for Life Ezekiel 4:9 Burger Bun (150) with 1 tablespoon **pesto** (80). Top with 3 ounces cooked/roasted chicken breast (122), a lettuce leaf (1), and 3 tomato slices (8).

  ▦ Total Calories = 361

Smoky Eggplant Wrap: Fill 1 Thomas' Sahara 100% Whole Wheat Wrap (170) with 3 tablespoons baba ghanoush (smoked eggplant) (120), ¼ cup diced seedless cucumber (4), 1 cup shredded lettuce (8), ¼ cup diced tomatoes (8), and 2 tablespoons **black olive tapenade** (88).

  ▦ Total Calories = 398

Beef and Gruyère Hoagie: Split 1 whole wheat hoagie (180) and cover both sides with 1 tablespoon **extra-virgin olive oil** (119). Brown in a nonstick skillet. Top with

2 ounces of all-natural top round roast beef (80), ½ ounce Gruyère cheese slice (58), and 1 teaspoon horseradish (2). Add vegetable toppings as desired.

  ▦ Total Calories = 439

Shredded Pork Pita: Fill 1 (6½") whole wheat pita (170) with 2 ounces cooked pulled or shredded pork (180). Warm in the microwave oven. Add 2 tablespoons **green olive tapenade** (54) and vegetable toppings as desired.

  ▦ Total Calories = 404

Easy Tuna Melt: Top 1 slice whole grain bread (80) with 4 ounces drained canned tuna (140), 1 ounce (1 slice) low-fat Colby cheese (48), and 1 tablespoon Hellman's **canola oil mayonnaise** (100). Toast in toaster oven and then add a lettuce leaf (1) and 3 tomato slices (8).

  ▦ Total Calories = 377

Refried Bean Wrap: Fill 1 Thomas' Sahara 100% Whole Wheat Wrap (170) with ½ cup Amy's Organic Refried Black Beans (140) and warm it in the oven or microwave oven. Top with 1 cup diced vegetables (30) and ¼ cup **Florida avocado** (69).

  ▦ Total Calories = 409

Bluesy Chicken Wraps: Stuff 2 large romaine lettuce leaves (2) equally with 3 ounces grilled chicken breast cubes or strips (122), 3 tablespoons blue cheese crumbles (75), 1/4 cup diced red and green bell peppers (7), 1/2 cup diced tomatoes (16), 2 tablespoons scallions (4), and liberal amounts of Frank's hot sauce. Serve with 2 tablespoons **Brazil nuts** (110) and 1 orange (69).

   Total Calories = 405

Chick-cran-stachio Salad: Combine 2 cups organic mixed baby greens (18), 3 ounces cooked/roasted chicken breast (122), 1 cup chopped vegetables of your choice (40), 1/8 cup dried cranberries (50), and 2 tablespoons **pistachios** (88). Dress with 1 tablespoon extra-virgin olive oil (119) and 2 tablespoons balsamic vinegar (10).

   Total Calories = 447

Meatball Melt: Fill 1 Thomas' Sahara Multi-Grain Pita (140) with 4 Trader Joe's Veggie Meatballs (93) and 2 tablespoons shredded part-skim mozzarella cheese (32). Drizzle with 1 tablespoon **extra-virgin olive oil** (119). Toast or broil to melt cheese. Serve with 1/4 cup Newman's Own Marinara Sauce (35) for dipping.

   Total Calories = 419

Chipotle Veggie Burger: Fill 1 whole grain burger bun (150) with a Gardenburger Black Bean Chipotle Veggie Burger (100), 1/4 cup **Hass avocado** (96), and 2 tablespoons Pace Pico de Gallo (10). Serve with 1 medium apple (77).

   Total Calories = 433

Chicken Lettuce Wraps: Fill 2 large romaine lettuce leaves (2) with 3 ounces grilled chicken breast (122) and brush with 2 tablespoons China Blue Scallion Ginger Glaze (80). Serve with a side of 1/2 cup fresh snow peas (20) and 2 tablespoons hummus (50) with 2 tablespoons **pine nuts** (113).

   Total Calories = 387

Boca Tacos: Warm 3 (6") corn tortillas (158) and fill with 1 cup warmed Boca Ground Burger Crumbles (120). Top with 1/2 cup fresh baby spinach leaves (3), 2 tablespoons salsa (20), and 1/4 cup sliced **Hass avocado** (96).

   Total Calories = 397

Fontina Beef Pita: Fill 1 (6 1/2") whole wheat pita (170) with 2 ounces all-natural top round roast beef (80), 1 ounce Fontina cheese (109), and 2 tablespoons **green olive tapenade** (54).

   Total Calories = 413

Shrimp and Brown Rice Bowl: Serve 4 ounces cooked frozen shrimp (120) and 1/4 cup **Florida avocado** chunks (69) on 1 cup cooked Uncle Ben's Ready Whole Grain Medley Brown and Wild Rice (220). Drizzle with 1 tablespoon reduced-sodium soy sauce (10).

   Total Calories = 419

Lunch Crudités: Top 1/2 cup hummus (200) with 2 tablespoons **pine nuts** (113) and serve with 1 cup celery strips (15), 1 cup baby carrots (53), and 1 cup broccoli florets (20).

   Total Calories = 401

Greek Tortilla Pizza: Top 1 Thomas' Sahara 100% Whole Wheat Wrap (170) with ½ cup Newman's Own Marinara Sauce (70), 1 ounce feta cheese (75), ½ cup cooked (fresh or frozen) spinach (21), and 10 sliced **large black olives** (50). Toast in a toaster oven.
▪ **Total Calories = 386**

Chilled Spicy Italian Sausage Pasta: Cook and chop 1 Applegate Farms Organic Sweet Italian Sausage (130). Toss with ¼ cup cooked and chilled whole wheat penne (105), 1 cup halved grape tomatoes (30), ¾ cup shredded carrots (38), ¼ cup chopped celery (5), and 1 tablespoon **pesto** (80).
▪ **Total Calories = 388**

Italian Sausage Wraps: Heat 1 tablespoon **canola oil** (124) in a nonstick pan and sauté 1 Applegate Farms Organic Sweet Italian Sausage, chopped (130), 1 cup fresh chopped bell pepper (28), and ½ cup sliced red onion (32). Spread evenly on 4 large romaine leaves (4), sprinkle with 2 tablespoons crumbed gorgonzola cheese (50), and roll up.
▪ **Total Calories = 368**

Gimme a Break

Eating lunch, just like exercise, doesn't magically happen unless you *make* it happen. Whether at work, at home, or in between, it's easy to fall victim to the myriad distractions: from the computer screen, to your phone, or your to-do list. You glance at the clock, and it's noon; then, suddenly it's 3:00 p.m. How'd that happen? Now, of course, you're ravenous, and fast food, fried food, or just about *any* food is impossible to resist. Instead of starving and then splurging, take some time to think about your meals and snacks beforehand. When will you have them? What will they look like? Where can you take 10 minutes to eat in peace and quiet, or at least without the bells and whistles of technology calling? Take the time to take a break and you will see a big difference in your weight loss results—guaranteed.

➜ Flat Belly Dinners

It's dinnertime! Whether you're a novice in the kitchen or an experienced gourmet, our Flat Belly dinners will help you lose weight and stay satisfied. As with the breakfasts and lunches, MUFAs are in **boldface,** and ingredient calorie counts are in parentheses.

Tex-Mex Soup: Heat 1 tablespoon **sunflower oil** (120) in a nonstick skillet. Add 3 ounces flank steak (158), ½ teaspoon minced garlic (2), ¼ cup diced tomatoes and onions (8), a dash of cumin, a dash of chili powder, and ¼ cup beef broth (4). Cook until beef is done and vegetables are tender. Top with 4 tablespoons low-fat shredded Cheddar cheese (80) and 5 baked tortilla chips, crumbled (50).
■ **Total Calories = 422**

Quick Chicken Casserole: Warm 3 ounces grilled/cooked chicken (122) in a pot with ½ cup low-sodium cream of chicken soup (120), ⅔ cup mixed frozen vegetables (50), 10 sliced large **black olives** (50), and ½ cup cooked whole wheat pasta (87).
■ **Total Calories = 429**

Blended Peanut Soup: Sauté ¼ cup chopped celery (4) and 2 tablespoons chopped onion (9) in 1 teaspoon olive oil (40) for 3 to 5 minutes or until soft. Add 1 cup reduced-sodium chicken broth (17), 1 teaspoon sherry vinegar (0), and 1 teaspoon lemon juice (1). Bring to a boil, then reduce heat and simmer for 5 to 7 minutes. Just before serving, stir in 2 tablespoons smooth **peanut butter** (188). Serve with 1 whole wheat pita (120).
■ **Total Calories = 379**

Turkey and Brie Quesadilla: Brush 1 Thomas' Sahara 100% Whole Wheat Wrap (170) with 1 tablespoon **sunflower oil** (120) and warm in a skillet. Top with 1 ounce brie (95) and 2 ounces sliced deli turkey (61).
■ **Total Calories = 446**

Southwest Potato: Microwave 1 medium baking potato (5.5 ounces) (161) for 5 to 6 minutes, then top with ¾ cup Amy's Organic Black Bean Chili (150), ¼ cup **Hass avocado** (96), and 1 tablespoon fat-free sour cream (8).
■ **Total Calories = 415**

Nanosecond Nachos: Arrange 12 baked tortilla chips (1 ounce) (118) on a plate and top with ¼ cup Kraft Natural Mexican Style Four Cheese (100) and ¼ cup pinto beans (61). Microwave to melt cheese. Add ¼ cup **Hass avocado** (96) and 1 cup diced tomatoes (32).
■ **Total Calories = 407**

Shredded "Beef" Burrito: Top 1 Thomas' Sahara 100% Whole Wheat Wrap (170) with 3 ounces warmed Lightlife Steak Style Strips (80), 2 tablespoons diced onions (6), 1 sliced jalapeño (4), 1 cup baby spinach leaves (24), and 10 sliced large **black olives** (50). Serve with 1 medium kiwifruit (46).
■ **Total Calorie = 380**

Slaw Dog: Heat 1 Lightlife Smart Dog (45) in the microwave oven. Place on 1 hot dog bun (170) with 1 tablespoon mustard (0) and 6 ounces Mann's Broccoli Cole Slaw (50) mixed with 1 tablespoon Hellman's **canola oil mayonnaise** (100).
■ Total Calories = 365

Mediterranean Sandwich: Mix 4 ounces chunk light water-packed tuna, drained (140), with 1 tablespoon Hellman's **canola oil mayonnaise** (100), 1 tablespoon rice vinegar (0), 1 teaspoon chopped parsley (0), and 1 teaspoon lemon juice (1). Serve between 2 slices of whole grain bread (160).
■ Total Calories = 406

Tomato and Mozzarella Salad: Combine 1 cup grape tomatoes (27), 3 ounces cherry-sized mozzarella balls (213), 1/4 cup fresh basil leaves (3), 1 tablespoon **extra-virgin olive oil** (119), 1 teaspoon balsamic vinegar (3), and black pepper to taste. Serve with half a toasted English muffin (68).
■ Total Calories = 433

Reuben Reduced: Combine 1/4 cup canned drained sauerkraut (7) and 1 tablespoon low-fat Thousand Island dressing (31). Slather onto 1 slice rye bread (63) and layer 3 ounces deli turkey (92) and 1 slice Swiss cheese (106). Heat 1 tablespoon **safflower oil** (120) in a skillet on medium to high heat and grill sandwich.
■ Total Calories = 419

Tuna Tacos: Marinate a 3-ounce tuna steak (123) in 1/2 teaspoon Worcestershire sauce (3). Microwave covered for approximately 3 minutes or until opaque. Then let fish stand 1 minute more. Mix 6 ounces Broccoli Cole Slaw (50) with 2 tablespoons Hellman's **canola oil mayonnaise** (100). Distribute tuna evenly over 3 (6") corn tortillas (158) and top with 1 tablespoon chopped red onion (4).
■ Total Calories = 438

Tuna and Avocado Sandwich: Drain a 5-ounce can chunk light tuna packed in water (175) and mix with 1/4 cup mashed **Hass avocado** (96). Spread on 2 slices of whole grain bread (160).
■ Total Calories = 431

Pepperoni Pizza: Brush 1 side of a Thomas' Sahara Multi-Grain Pita (140) with 1 tablespoon **extra-virgin olive oil** (119) and top with 1/2 cup Newman's Own Marinara Sauce (70), 13 slices Lightlife Smart Deli Pepperoni (50), and 2 tablespoons Organic Valley Shredded Italian Blend (45). Warm under the broiler or in a toaster oven to heat through and melt cheese.
■ Total Calories = 424

Savory Turkey Pasta: Sauté 1/2 cup broccoli florets (20) and 1 cup sliced plum tomatoes (30) in 1 tablespoon **sunflower oil** (120) and toss with 4 fresh basil leaves, sliced (0), 3 ounces browned all-breast-meat ground turkey (90), and 1/4 cup cooked whole wheat penne (105).
■ Total Calories = 365

Szechuan Chicken: Sauté 2 cups frozen Cascadian Farm Organic Chinese Stirfry Mixed Vegetables (50) in 1 tablespoon **canola oil** (124) flavored with ground Szechuan peppercorns. Serve with 4 ounces organic grilled chicken breast (120) and ½ cup cooked Uncle Ben's Ready Rice Whole Grain Brown (120).

　▪ **Total Calories = 414**

Dijon Basil Chicken: Rub 5 ounces chicken breast (203) with 1 teaspoon Dijon mustard (5) and cook in 1 tablespoon **extra-virgin olive oil** (119) with 5 sliced basil leaves (0). Serve with 1 cup steamed green beans (34) and 1 medium peach (59).

　▪ **Total Calories = 420**

Curried Pork Stir-Fry: Cut 4 ounces pork loin into strips (132) and sprinkle with ¼ teaspoon curry powder (0). Cook with 1 cup snow peas (26) in 1 tablespoon **sesame oil** (120) for 4 to 5 minutes. Serve with ½ cup cooked Uncle Ben's Ready Whole Grain Medley Brown and Wild Rice (110).

　▪ **Total Calories = 388**

Chicken Caesar Salad: Marinate 5 ounces chicken breast (203) in 2 tablespoons Kraft Caesar Vinaigrette with Parmesan (70), then grill for 5 minutes. Place chicken atop 3 cups shredded romaine lettuce (24) and top with 1 tablespoon shredded Parmesan cheese (21), 1 tablespoon **extra-virgin olive oil** (119), and 2 anchovies for garnish (16).

　▪ **Total Calories = 453**

Parmesan Pork Chop: Dredge a 5-ounce boneless pork chop (200) in 2 tablespoons Progresso Parmesan Bread Crumbs (50) and cook in 1 tablespoon **sunflower oil** (120) for 5 minutes. Serve with 1 cup steamed zucchini slices (25).

　▪ **Total Calories = 395**

Honey-Glazed Salmon: Brush a 4-ounce salmon fillet (233) with 1 tablespoon Kraft Honey Mustard Barbecue Sauce (40) and cook in a 325°F oven until the fish flakes easily with a fork. Serve with 1 cup steamed asparagus (27) drizzled with 1 tablespoon **walnut oil** (120) and the juice of 1 lemon wedge (2).

　▪ **Total Calories = 422**

Halibut Italiano: Brush 6 ounces halibut (186) with 2 tablespoons Kraft Caesar Vinaigrette with Parmesan (70) and topped with 1 tablespoon scallions (2). Cover and microwave for 2 minutes. Let fish stand 1 minute. Steam 1 cup Italian blend vegetables (40) with 2 tablespoons slivered **almonds** (109).

　▪ **Total Calories = 407**

Southwest Quick Shrimp: Toss 3 cups chopped romaine lettuce (24), 5 ounces cooked shrimp (140), ¼ cup **Hass avocado** (96), ¼ cup corn kernels (40), 1 cup grape tomatoes (27), 2 baked tortilla chips, crumbled (20), and 2 tablespoons reduced-fat ranch dressing (66).

　▪ **Total Calories = 413**

Mushroom Caps: Brush 2 portobello mushroom caps (3 ounces each) (44) with 1 tablespoon **peanut oil** (119) and 2 tablespoons balsamic vinegar (10) and grill. Serve with 1 cup steamed green beans (34), ½ cup cooked Uncle Ben's Ready Rice Whole Grain Brown (120), and 1 small pear (86).

◼ **Total Calories = 413**

Spicy Omelet Scramble: Whisk 2 large eggs (143) and cook as an omelet in a skillet with 1 tablespoon **canola oil** (124). Top with ½ cup rinsed and drained black beans (100) and 4 tablespoons Pace Pico de Gallo (20). Fold and serve.

◼ **Total Calories = 387**

MESSAGE FROM MILTON

Protein: How Much Is Enough?

Every guy I counsel in my practice is concerned about getting enough protein. Fact is, most are already getting more than enough. From meat to milk to whole grains, protein is just about everywhere. A simple calculation can help you determine your protein needs for the day: Multiply 0.8 gram of protein per kilogram of your body weight. So, let's say you weigh 190 pounds. Convert pounds to kilograms by dividing 190 by 2.2 = 86.4. Then multiply that by 0.8 = 69 grams protein. (A typical quarter-pound hamburger has about 28 grams of protein in the meat alone. Add cheese and a bun and you're up to 35 or more.) The average guy already consumes much more than that. (If you are a bodybuilder, protein needs are only slightly higher: 1.3 to 1.7 grams per kilogram of body weight.) The question is, are you getting the *right* kinds of protein? The Colonel's Secret Recipe Chicken, for example, has lots of protein, but it's also packed with lots of artery-clogging saturated fat. Choose your protein wisely. Think lean cuts of beef, pork, and poultry; fatty fish; beans, hummus, and nuts; and low-fat or fat-free dairy products. The Flat Belly recipes, quick meals, and restaurant guide will help you make healthier protein choices.

→ Flat Belly Power Snacks

No need to give up snacking to lose weight! These snacks will power you through your day without a grumbling stomach. Again, MUFAs are in **boldface,** and ingredient calorie counts are in parentheses.

Savory

Ginger Tahini Dip with Crudité:

Combine 2 tablespoons **tahini** (178) with 1 teaspoon chopped fresh cilantro (0), 1 teaspoon toasted sesame oil (33), 1 teaspoon honey (20), and ¼ teaspoon ground ginger (0) as a dip for 1 cup sliced red bell pepper (28). Serve with 1 medium pear (103) and 1 Laughing Cow Garlic and Herb Wedge (35).
■ **Total Calories = 397**

Triscuit MUFA Minis: Spread

2 tablespoons **black olive tapenade** (88) on 7 Triscuit Fire Roasted Tomato and Olive Oil Crackers (140). Top with 1 (½-ounce) Muenster cheese slice (155). Warm in the microwave oven for 30 seconds.
■ **Total Calories = 383**

Nutty Cottage Cheese: Top 1 cup

low-fat (1% milk) cottage cheese (162) with 2 cups melon balls (120) and 2 tablespoons **hazelnuts** (110).
■ **Total Calories = 392**

Pita Chips and Tapenade: Serve

1 ounce (about 6) Athenos Roasted Garlic and Herb pita chips (120) with 2 tablespoons **black olive tapenade** (88) for dipping. Serve with ½ cup dried apricots (157) on the side.
■ **Total Calories = 365**

Spiced Edamame: Mix 1 cup shelled

and boiled **edamame** (244) with ¼ teaspoon ground cumin (0) and 1 dash cayenne pepper (0). Serve with ¾ cup cooked brown rice (164).
■ **Total Calories = 408**

Pesto Baked Potato: Microwave

1 medium baking potato (5.5 ounces) (145) for 5 minutes, then top with 1 tablespoon **pesto** (80), ½ cup low-fat (1% milk) cottage cheese (81), and 2 tablespoons fat-free sour cream (16). Serve with 1 cup grapes (104) on the side.
■ **Total Calories = 426**

Pesto Turkey Rollup: Layer

4 ounces deli turkey meat (122) with 2 ounces baby Swiss (200) and 1 tablespoon **pesto** (80). Roll and slice.
■ **Total Calories = 402**

Cheese, Nuts, and Fruit: Serve 2

Horizon Organic Colby Cheese Sticks (220) with 2 tablespoons **cashews** (100) and ¼ cup dried cranberries (104).
■ **Total Calories = 424**

PB Vegged Out: Dip 1 cup baby car-

rots (53) and 1 cup celery sticks (15) in 2 tablespoons smooth **peanut butter** (188). Serve with 1 cup fat-free milk (83).
■ **Total Calories = 339**

Sweet

Open-Faced PB and Honey:

Spread 1 slice whole grain bread (70) with
2 tablespoons crunchy **peanut butter** (188)
and top with 1 sliced banana (105). Drizzle
with 1 teaspoon honey (20).

■ Total Calories = 383

Waffle Sundae: Toast 1 Nature's Path

Organic Flax Plus Frozen Waffle (90), then top
with 1/2 cup Breyers Natural Vanilla Ice Cream
(130), 1 sliced kiwifruit (46), and 2 tablespoons
crushed **macadamia nuts** (120).

■ Total Calories = 386

PB Sundae: Heat 2 tablespoons smooth

peanut butter (188) in the microwave oven for
30 seconds, then drizzle over 1/2 cup Breyers
Natural Vanilla Ice Cream (130). Top with
1 tablespoon Hershey's chocolate syrup (50).

■ Total Calories = 368

Cake Sundae: Top 1 slice of pound cake

(1/12 of average cake; 1 ounce) (109) with 1 cup
fruit cocktail in its own juice (110) and 2 tablespoons **walnuts** (82). Serve with 1 cup fat-free
milk (83).

■ Total Calories = 384

S'mores: Layer 1/4 cup semisweet choco-

late chips (207) and 40 miniature marshmal-
lows (88) on 2 large rectangular graham
cracker pieces (120). Microwave to warm
throughout, about 30 to 45 seconds.

■ Total Calories = 415

Mini Decadent Feast: Serve 1/4 cup

semisweet chocolate chips (207) with
1 ounce Camembert cheese (100) and
2 dried figs (94).

■ Total Calories = 401

Yogurt Crunch Delight: Mix 1 cup

(8 ounces) fat-free plain Stonyfield Farm
Oikos Organic Greek Yogurt (130) with
2 tablespoons **sunflower seeds** (90). Drizzle
1 tablespoon honey (64) on top. Serve with
1 banana (105) on the side.

■ Total Calories = 389

Cereal Break: Serve 3/4 cup Nature's

Path Organic Flax Plus Red Berry Crunch
cereal (220) with 1 cup fat-free milk (83) and
2 tablespoons **walnuts** (82).

■ Total Calories = 385

Italian Power Snack: Roll 1 1/2 ounces

prosciutto (122) around 1 cup honeydew
melon (64). Serve with 1 ounce provolone
cheese (100) and 2 tablespoons **almonds**
(109).

■ Total Calories = 395

Trail Mix: Combine 2 tablespoons sun-

flower seeds (90), 2 tablespoons semisweet
chocolate chips (140), 1 ounce Rold Gold Tiny
Twists Pretzels (110), and 1 miniature box of
raisins (30 raisins, 0.5 ounce) (42).

■ Total Calories = 382

Grab & Go

Option 1: 2 low-fat string cheese (160), 1 pineapple fruit cup (in its own juice) (59), 1 cup baby carrots (53), and 2 tablespoons **peanuts** (110).
- Total Calories = 382

Option 2: 2 low-fat string cheese (160), 4 cups popped light microwave popcorn (100), 1/4 cup grated Parmesan cheese (88), and 2 tablespoons **sunflower seeds** (90).
- Total Calories = 438

Option 3: 6 ounces Stonyfield Farm Fat-Free French Vanilla Yogurt (130), 1 apple (77), 2 tablespoons **Brazil nuts (110)**, and 1 cup fat-free milk (83).
- Total Calories = 400

Smoothies

Peanut Butter–Banana: Blend 1 medium banana (105), 2 tablespoons natural smooth **peanut butter** (188), 6 ounces fat-free plain Greek yogurt (90), 1/4 cup fat-free milk (21), 1/4 teaspoon vanilla extract (3), dash of cinnamon (0), and 1/4 cup ice (0) for 1 minute. Transfer to a glass.
- Total Calories = 409

Tropical: Blend 1/2 cup soft tofu (75), 8 ounces 100% pineapple fruit juice (146), 1/4 cup mango (fresh or frozen) (54), and 1/4 cup ice (0) for 1 minute. Transfer to a glass. Garnish with 2 tablespoons chopped **pistachios** (88).
- Total calories = 363

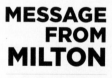

MESSAGE FROM MILTON

Got the Munchies?

Eating too little throughout the day guarantees hunger will strike the moment you set foot in the door. With your mind no longer occupied by the daily grind, you'll be on the prowl for snack foods. Chances are you'll be ready to grab and gobble just about anything. However, if you eat adequately during the workday—at least three 400-calorie meals—this will minimize ravenous eating at the end of the day. And if you eat a good-for-you Power Snack instead of grabbing whatever is close at hand, you'll fill up but not out. The snack options beginning on page 130 comprise healthy carbs, the right amount of protein, and that magic MUFA, making them a balanced way to tame the munchie monster.

Melon Morning: Blend 1 cup watermelon balls (46), 1 cup cantaloupe balls (60), 1 cup honeydew balls (64), 6 ounces Stonyfield Farm Fat-Free French Vanilla Yogurt (130), 1 tablespoon **flaxseed oil** (120), and ¼ cup ice for 1 minute. Transfer to a glass.
■ **Total Calories = 420**

Apple Pie: Blend 6 ounces Stonyfield Farm Fat-Free French Vanilla Yogurt (130), 1 teaspoon apple pie spice (0), 1 medium apple, peeled, cored, and chopped (77), 2 tablespoons **almond butter** (200), and a handful of ice for 1 minute. Transfer to a glass.
■ **Total Calories = 407**

Banana Chocolate: Blend 1 banana (105), ½ cup fat-free milk (42), 2 tablespoons unsweetened cocoa powder (25), 2 teaspoons honey (40), 2 tablespoons **cashew butter** (190), and a handful of ice for 1 minute. Transfer to a glass.
■ **Total Calories = 402**

Berries and Cream: Blend ½ cup Breyers Natural Vanilla Ice Cream (130), 1 cup raspberries (64), 1 tablespoon **walnut oil** (120), 1 cup fat-free milk (83), and a handful of ice for 1 minute. Transfer to a glass.
■ **Total Calories = 397**

Make Your Own Meals + Power Snacks

REMEMBER YOUR TARGET IS 400 CALORIES. ENSURE EACH MEAL OR SNACK COMPRISES A MUFA FROM THE LIST ON PAGE 99 PAIRED WITH SOME OF THE FOLLOWING:

SOME MUFA CHOICES:

- 10 olives
- 1 cup soybeans
- ¼ cup avocado
- ¼ cup semisweet chocolate chips
- 2 tablespoons nuts or seeds
- 2 tablespoons olive tapenade
- 1 tablespoon oil

Please consult the full chart on page 99

GRAINS

Corn tortillas (2), 105 calories

Food For Life Ezekiel 4:9 Organic Sesame Sprouted Grain Bread (1 slice), 80 calories

Nature's Path Organic Flax Plus Frozen Waffle (1), 90 calories

Oatmeal (1 packet, 1 ounce) instant, plain, 100 calories

Popcorn (4 cups popped; Smart Balance Light or Newman's Own 94% fat-free), 100 calories

Thomas' Sahara Multi-Grain Pita (½ pita), 70 calories

Thomas' Hearty Grains 100% Whole Wheat Bagel (½), 135 calories

Thomas' Hearty Grains 100% Whole Wheat English Muffin (1 whole), 120 calories

Thomas' Sahara 100% Whole Wheat Wrap (1 whole), 170 calories

Uncle Ben's Ready Rice Whole Grain Brown (½ cup), 120 calories

DAIRY

Applegate Farms Organic Monterey Jack with Jalapeño Peppers (1 slice), 80 calories

Cottage cheese, fat-free (½ cup), 81 calories

Kraft Natural Mexican Style Four Cheese (¼ cup), 100 calories

Milk, fat-free (1 cup) 83 calories

Organic Valley Shredded Italian Blend (¼ cup), 90 calories

Stonyfield Farm Fat-Free French Vanilla Yogurt (6 ounces), 130 calories

Stonyfield Farm Oikos Organic Greek Yogurt, fat-free plain (8 ounces), 130 calories

String cheese, low-fat (1 ounce), 80 calories

Yogurt, plain fat-free (6 ounces), 80 calories

FRUITS

Apple, any variety, medium (size of a tennis ball), 77 calories

Banana (medium), 105 calories

Blueberries (1 cup), 84 calories

Grapes (1 cup), 104 calories

Mango (1 cup sliced), 110 calories

Mott's Natural Unsweetened Apple Sauce (1 cup), 100 calories

Orange (medium), 69 calories

Peach (medium), 59 calories

Pineapple, canned in pineapple juice (4 ounces or ½ cup), 59 calories

Raisins, unsweetened (¼ cup), 123 calories

Raspberries (1 cup), 64 calories

Strawberries (1 cup), 54 calories

Watermelon (2 cups diced), 92 calories

VEGETABLES

Artichoke hearts, canned in water (1 cup), 90 calories

Baba ghanoush (smoked eggplant spread, 2 tablespoons), 80 calories

Baby carrots (1 cup), 53 calories

Baked potato (medium, 5.5 ounces), 161 calories

Broccoli florets, raw (2 cups), 40 calories

Grape tomatoes (1 cup), 30 calories

Mann's Broccoli Cole Slaw (12-ounce bag), 100 calories

Newman's Own Marinara Sauce (½ cup), 70 calories

Mixed baby field greens (2 cups), 18 calories

Red bell pepper, sliced (1 cup), 28 calories

Salsa (¼ cup), 20 calories

PROTEINS

Black Forest ham (4 ounces), 122 calories

Black beans, canned, drained (½ cup), 100 calories

Chicken breast, precooked (3 ounces), 122 calories

Chunk light tuna in water (3 ounces), 105 calories

Deli turkey slices (4 ounces), 122 calories

Egg, large (1), 78 calories

Gardenburger Black Bean Chipotle Veggie Burger, 100 calories

Trader Joe's Veggie Meatballs (6), 140 calories

Ground beef, 95% extra-lean, cooked (4 ounces), 193 calories

Hummus (¼ cup), 100 calories

Pork tenderloin, roasted (3 ounces), 99 calories

Flat Belly Diet Ready-Made Meals

THE MEALS AND POWER SNACKS in this plan make it easy for you to follow the Flat Belly Diet for Men rules when you have the time to plan ahead and make your meals. But what about those times when you're traveling or stuck in the office and you forgot to bring your Flat Belly Diet meals? Here, you'll find recommendations for specific brand-name products, which *Prevention* magazine has screened to make sure they're free of trans fats and artificial sweeteners and which can provide a great shortcut for meals and snacks when you're short on time. You'll also find lists of Flat Belly Diet–friendly entrées on the menus of popular national restaurant and fast-food chains. These are great options when you're in a pinch, but, ultimately, you should pick these no more than once or twice a day.

MESSAGE FROM MILTON

You Are What You Drink

An extra 140 calories here, 240 there. That's what drinking, but not thinking, can result in. Regular soda, sugar-sweetened teas, coffee with cream and sugar, and beer—liquid calories add up fast. And we rarely compensate for those extra calories by eating less food. Time and time again I see clients who live off sports drinks. At 50 calories per cup, that's a surefire way to undo any weight loss progress. You'd have to mountain bike at least 20 minutes to burn off the calories from a typical bottle of a sports drink. Instead, eat your calories in the form of real food and drink water or unsweetened beverages. Weight will drop a lot faster, and you won't miss the sugary syrup.

MEAL REPLACEMENT BARS

CHOOSE 1 OF THE FOLLOWING MEAL REPLACEMENT BARS	CALORIES	ADD YOUR MUFA
Clif Black Cherry Almond Bar	250	
Clif Crunchy Peanut Butter Bar	250	
PowerBar HARVEST Oatmeal Raisin Cookie	250	
PowerBar HARVEST Toffee Chocolate Chip	250	Add 1 piece of fruit and a 100- to 150-calorie MUFA from the list on page 99, such as 2 tablespoons of (choose one):
Clif Chocolate Brownie Bar	240	
Nature's Path Optimum Pomegran Cherry Energy Bar	230	
Larabar Chocolate Coconut	220	
Larabar Banana Bread	220	almonds (109)
Larabar Ginger Snap	220	Brazil nuts (110)
Odwalla Banana Nut Bar	220	peanuts (110)
Larabar Cinnamon Roll	210	macadamia nuts (120)
Odwalla Choco-walla Bar	210	
Nature's Path Optimum Blueberry Flax & Soy Energy Bar	200	OR
Larabar Pecan Pie	200	Add a 150- to 200-calorie MUFA from the list such as 2 tablespoons of (choose one):
Larabar Cherry Pie	190	
Kashi GOLEAN Crunchy! Chocolate Peanut Bar	180	
Larabar Apple Pie	180	natural peanut butter (188)
Kashi GOLEAN Crunchy! Chocolate Almond Bar	170	almond butter (200)
Kashi GOLEAN Crunchy! Chocolate Caramel Bar	150	
Kellogg's Fiber Plus Dark Chocolate Almond Bar	130	
Kellogg's Fiber Plus Chocolate Chip Bar	120	

FROZEN MEALS

CHOOSE 1 OF THE FOLLOWING MEALS	CALORIES	ADD YOUR MUFA
Amy's Chili and Cornbread Whole Meal	340	
Kashi Black Bean Mango	340	
Amy's Black Bean Enchilada Whole Meal	330	
Amy's Indian Mattar Paneer	320	
Kashi Sweet and Sour Chicken	320	
Seeds of Change Fettuccine Alfredo di Roma	320	Add a 50- to 100-calorie MUFA from the list on page 99, such as:
Amy's Indian Vegetable Korma	310	
Kashi Lemongrass Coconut Chicken	300	10 large green or black olives (or 5 of each) (50)
Seeds of Change Hanalei Vegetarian Chicken Teriyaki	300	
Amy's Organic Brown Rice, Black-Eyed Peas & Veggies Bowl	290	
Amy's Organic Teriyaki Bowl	290	
Amy's Veggie Loaf Whole Meal	290	
Boca Lasagna with Chunky Tomato and Herb Sauce	290	
Kashi Chicken Florentine	290	
Kashi Chicken Pasta Pomodoro	280	Add a 100- to 150-calorie MUFA from the list on page 99, such as 2 tablespoons of (choose 1):
Seeds of Change Lasagna Calabrese with Eggplant and Portobello Mushrooms	270	
Amy's Indian Mattar Tofu	260	almonds (109) peanuts (110)
Kashi Southwest Style Chicken	240	pumpkin seeds (148)
Cedarlane Low Fat Veggie Pizza Wrap	220	Add a 150- to 200-calorie MUFA from the list on page 99, such as:
Yves Veggie Penne	210	
Amy's Light in Sodium Shepherd's Pie	160	
Boca Meatless Chili	150	¼ cup chocolate chips (207)

FAST FOOD

MENU ITEM(S)	CALORIES	ADD YOUR MUFA
McDonald's Premium Southwest Salad with Grilled Chicken and Newman's Own Lighten Up Italian Dressing	380	Add a 50- to 100-calorie MUFA from the list on page 99, such as:
Taco Bell Fresco Bean Burrito	340	
Jack in the Box Asian Grilled Chicken Salad with Roasted Slivered Almonds and Low-Fat Balsamic Dressing	325	☐ 10 large green or black olives (or 5 of each) (50)
Baja Fresh Baja Ensalada with Charbroiled Chicken with Fat-Free Salsa Verde	310	☐ 2 tablespoons walnuts (82)
Au Bon Pain Southwest Vegetable Soup (medium) with Cheddar Jalapeño Breadstick	300	☐ 2 tablespoons pistachios (89)
Pizza Hut Fit n' Delicious Pizza (2 slices) with Green Pepper, Red Onion & Diced Tomato (12")	300	☐ 2 tablespoons sunflower seeds (90)
Boston Market Roasted Turkey Breast with Poultry Gravy and Steamed Vegetables	290	
Panda Express String Bean Chicken Breast with Mixed Vegetables	290	Add a 100- to 150-calorie MUFA from the list on page 99, such as:
Arby's Junior Roast Beef Sandwich	270	
Fazoli's Chicken and Artichoke Salad with Fat-Free Italian Dressing	265	☐ 2 tablespoons pumpkin seeds (148)
Chick-fil-A Chargrilled Chicken Sandwich	260	
Panera Low-Fat Vegetarian Garden Vegetable Soup with a Whole Grain Loaf	260	
Subway Oven Roasted Chicken Salad with Fat-Free Italian Dressing and Roasted Chicken Noodle Soup	245	Add a 150- to 200-calorie MUFA from the list on page 99, such as 2 tablespoons of (choose 1):
Domino's Grilled Chicken Caesar with Light Italian Dressing and one breadstick	236	
Jamba Juice Blackberry Bliss Smoothie (16 ounces)	230	☐ natural peanut butter (188)
Wendy's Small Chili	190	
Taco Bell Ranchero Chicken Soft Taco (Fresco Style)	180	☐ almond butter (200)

READ A FLAT BELLY
SUCCESS
STORY

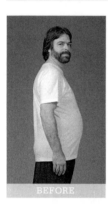

BEFORE

AFTER

Nelson Duran

AGE: 46

POUNDS LOST:

10.8

IN 32 DAYS

ALL-OVER
INCHES LOST:

7.25

3 FROM
THE WAIST

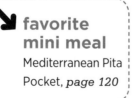

↘ **favorite
mini meal**
Mediterranean Pita
Pocket, *page 120*

When Nelson, the 46-year-old owner of a video production business in New York, came in for his final weigh-in, he had lots of changes to share. Yes, he lost a hefty amount of weight and inches, but he also reported that during the time he was on the test panel, his company went from near collapse to explosively busy, he sold his house, and he moved. He was one busy man. And he says he's never felt better.

"My struggle with weight stems from my addictive personality," says Nelson. "I often use food as a crutch in difficult or stressful times." But unlike other diets Nelson had tried in the past, he found the Flat Belly Diet for Men a breeze. "Other diets were difficult to follow because of the ratios of fat to protein to carbs," says Nelson. The number crunching and calorie counting left him frustrated. By the time he was ready to sit down and eat, he would be fed up and then just give up. "I didn't have time to calculate ratios all through the day."

Nelson found the MUFA Meal Plan helped him balance his meals and reduce his calories; NO number crunching required! "This was the easiest diet I've ever followed. And it wasn't even a diet. I had real food— and real food I actually like to eat." Real MUFA foods, that is. "The MUFAs made my meals interesting, like there was an added bonus every time I ate. And since the food tastes good, the plan is easy to follow." Nelson also appreciated the long list of Flat Belly–approved quick and frozen prepared meals. "I just never ran out of options."

In addition to the MUFA meals, Nelson credits some of his success to the Fire Water. "There's something about the hot sauce that curbed my appetite. And I felt it gave me a metabolism boost, too." Nelson prepared large batches of the water in advance that he kept in sports bottles so they were chilled and ready to go.

So, even with an overload of work stress and an entire household move, it's no wonder Nelson dropped nearly 11 pounds and 7.25 inches in just 4 weeks. "It never felt like a diet. It felt like life made easy."

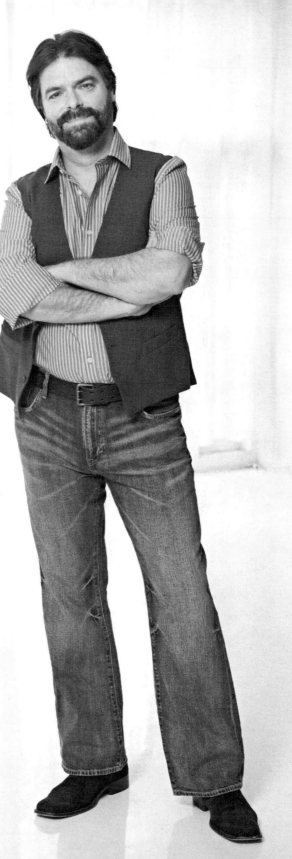

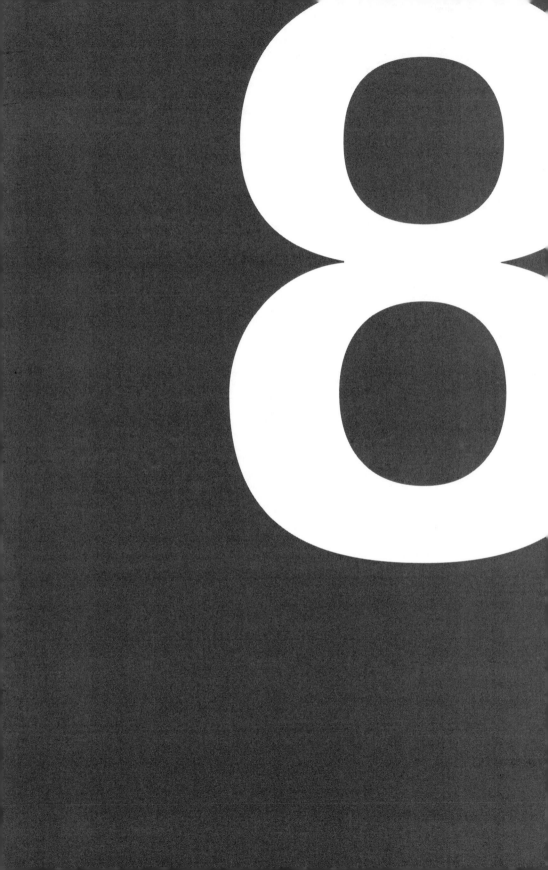

FLAT BELLY DIET MEN IN THE KITCHEN AND AT THE GRILL

THE RECIPES YOU'LL find here can be prepared regardless of your kitchen skills (or in my case, *lack* of kitchen skills). They're also so incredibly flavorful they'll make your mouth water. And the best thing about them is that they fit easily into the Flat Belly Diet for Men. Each serving contains a MUFA, for starters. As you know, MUFAs are the only foods that can specifically help reduce belly fat. You can spot them in the ingredient lists; they're in **boldface**. In addition, beside most recipes is a very important component titled "Make It a Flat Belly Diet Meal." This box tells you what to add to one serving of that recipe to turn it into a meal that you can slot right into your menu plan. And remember, the numbers in parentheses refer to the calorie counts of specific ingredients.

Don't worry. It's easier than it sounds! Let's get cooking!

RECIPE INDEX

■ ON THE GRILL (PAGES 178–189)

Monterey Jack and Jalapeño Turkey
   Burgers with Special Sauce
Grilled Chicken Breasts with Peanut
   Barbecue Sauce
Grilled Chicken Thighs with Avocado
   Salsa
Pesto-Parmesan-Topped Burgers on
   Portuguese Rolls
Grilled Flank Steak with Olive Oil Mojo
   Sauce
Grilled Filet Mignon with Grilled Onion
   and Avocado
Marinated Grilled Boneless Pork Ribs
Mediterranean-Style Lamb Chops with
   Cucumber Salad
Lemon-Herb-Marinated Tuna Burger with
   Wasabi Aioli
Asian-Marinated Grilled Tuna Steaks with
   Crunchy Peanut Dressing
Grilled Salmon with Herbs, Dijon, and
   Extra-Virgin Olive Oil
Balsamic Portobello and Vegetable
   Mixed Grill

■ POWER SNACKS & SIDES (PAGES 190–192)

Chili-Spiced Fries with Chipotle Ketchup
Mexican Bean and Avocado Salsa with
   Baked Tortilla Chips
Sautéed Spinach with Garlic and Red-
   Pepper Flakes

■ DESSERTS (PAGES 193–197)

Macadamia Nut Blondies
Dark Chocolate Pudding
Cashew Chocolate Chip Cookie Ice
   Cream Sandwiches
Strawberry-Banana and Pecan Sundaes
Cinnamon Apple Crisp

Almond, Blueberry, and Brown Sugar Oatmeal

Preparation time: 2 minutes / Cooking time: 5 minutes / Makes 4 servings

MUFA: ½ cup slivered almonds, toasted

2 cups 1% milk
1 cup oatmeal
3 tablespoons packed light brown sugar
½ teaspoon pure vanilla extract
¼ teaspoon salt
⅛ teaspoon ground nutmeg
1 cup fresh blueberries

1. Toast the almonds in a large nonstick skillet over medium heat, stirring often, for 3 to 4 minutes or until lightly browned and fragrant. Transfer to a plate and cool.

2. Combine the milk, oatmeal, sugar, vanilla, salt, and nutmeg in a medium saucepan over medium heat. Bring to a simmer and cook, stirring occasionally, 5 minutes or until oatmeal is tender. Stir in the blueberries and sprinkle with almonds.

■ **Eat One Serving:**

302

CALORIES,
11 g protein, 39 g carbohydrates, 12 g fat, 1.9 g saturated fat, 6 mg cholesterol, 212 mg sodium, 5 g fiber

MAKE IT A FLAT BELLY DIET MEAL:
Add 1 cup orange juice (112).

■ **Total Meal:**

414

CALORIES

Scrambled Breakfast Tacos with Chunky Guacamole

Preparation time: 10 minutes / Cooking time: 5 minutes / Makes 4 servings

MUFA: 1 Hass avocado, peeled, pitted, and diced

1 plum tomato, chopped

$\frac{1}{4}$ small white onion, chopped

1 tablespoon chopped fresh cilantro

$\frac{1}{2}$ teaspoon salt

4 eggs

4 egg whites

2 ounces shredded 50% reduced-fat sharp Cheddar cheese

$\frac{1}{4}$ teaspoon black pepper

1 teaspoon olive oil

8 corn tortillas

1. Combine the avocado, tomato, onion, cilantro, and $\frac{1}{4}$ teaspoon salt in a bowl.

2. Whisk together the eggs, egg whites, cheese, remaining $\frac{1}{4}$ teaspoon salt, and pepper in a bowl. Heat the oil in a medium nonstick skillet over medium-high heat. Add the egg mixture and cook, stirring occasionally, 3 to 4 minutes, or until set.

3. Heat the tortillas over a gas burner, turning occasionally, about 1 minute, or place the tortillas between clean paper towels and microwave on high for 15 to 20 seconds to warm. To serve, fill each with some of the egg mixture and top with the avocado mixture.

■ **Eat One Serving:**

335

CALORIES,
17 g protein, 33 g carbohydrates, 16 g fat, 3.9 g saturated fat, 212 mg cholesterol, 575 mg sodium, 5 g fiber

MAKE IT A FLAT BELLY DIET MEAL:
Add 1 cup reduced-sodium tomato juice (50).

■ **Total Meal:**

385

CALORIES

BREAKFAST

Ham and Tomato Omelet with Basil Pesto

Preparation time: 5 minutes / Cooking time: 5 minutes / Makes 2 servings

1 teaspoon olive oil
2 ounces deli sliced Virginia ham, chopped
¼ onion, finely chopped
2 eggs
4 egg whites

MUFA: 2 tablespoons basil pesto

½ cup shredded reduced-fat mozzarella cheese
1 plum tomato, seeded and chopped

1. Heat the oil in a medium nonstick skillet over medium-high heat. Add the ham and onion. Cook, stirring occasionally, for 3 to 4 minutes, or until starting to brown. Whisk together the egg, egg whites, and 1 tablespoon pesto in a medium bowl. Pour into the skillet.

2. Cook about 3 minutes, until the eggs begin to set in the center, using a silicone spatula to lift the set edges and allow the uncooked mixture to run underneath.

3. Scatter the cheese and tomato over half of the omelet. Cover and cook for 2 minutes or until just set. Spread the remaining 1 tablespoon pesto down the center of the omelet. Carefully loosen the omelet with the spatula and fold in half. Let rest 1 minute or until the cheese melts. Cut in half to serve.

■ Eat One Serving:

298

CALORIES,
24 g protein, 6 g carbohydrates, 20 g fat, 4.9 g saturated fat*, 6 mg cholesterol, 652 mg sodium*, 1 g fiber

MAKE IT A FLAT BELLY DIET MEAL:
Serve with a toasted whole grain English muffin (135).

■ Total Meal:

433

CALORIES

* Limit saturated fat to no more than 10% of total calories—about 20 grams for most men— and sodium intake to no more than 2,300 milligrams.

Rancho-Chipotle Omelet

Preparation time: 5 minutes / Cooking time: 5 minutes / Makes 2 servings

1 teaspoon olive oil
2 eggs
4 egg whites
¼ teaspoon salt
⅛ teaspoon black pepper
2 ounces shredded 50% reduced-fat sharp Cheddar cheese

MUFA: ½ Hass avocado, sliced

¼ cup prepared chipotle salsa
4 corn tortillas

1. Heat the oil in a medium nonstick skillet over medium-high heat.

2. Whisk together the eggs, egg whites, salt, and pepper in a medium bowl. Pour into the skillet.

3. Cook about 3 minutes until the eggs begin to set in the center, using a silicone spatula to lift up the set edges and allow the uncooked mixture to run underneath.

4. Scatter the cheese over half of the omelet. Cover and cook for 2 minutes or until just set. Top half of the omelet with the avocado and salsa. Carefully loosen the omelet with the spatula and fold in half. Let rest 1 minute or until the cheese melts. Heat the tortillas over a gas burner, turning occasionally, about 1 minute, or place the tortillas between clean paper towels and microwave on high for 15 to 20 seconds to warm. Cut the omelet in half and serve with the tortillas.

■ **Eat One Serving:**

366

CALORIES,
25 g protein, 28 g carbohydrates, 19 g fat, 6.8 g saturated fat*, 212 mg cholesterol, 792 mg sodium*, 5 g fiber

MAKE IT A FLAT BELLY DIET MEAL:
Add 1 cup of honeydew melon balls (64 calories).

■ **Total Meal:**

430

CALORIES

* Limit saturated fat to no more than 10% of total calories—about 20 grams for most men— and sodium intake to no more than 2,300 milligrams.

BREAKFAST

English Muffin Egg Sandwich with Spinach and Canadian Bacon

Preparation time: 10 minutes / Cooking time: 6 minutes / Makes 4 servings

2 teaspoons olive oil

4 cups baby spinach

MUFA: ¼ cup sun-dried tomato pesto

4 eggs

⅛ teaspoon black pepper

4 multigrain 100-calorie English muffins, toasted

4 slices Canadian bacon

1. Heat 1 teaspoon of the oil in a large nonstick skillet over medium-high heat. Add the spinach and cook, turning, about 1 minute, until wilted. Stir in 3 tablespoons pesto and cook 15 seconds. Transfer to a bowl and keep warm.

2. Return the skillet to the stove and heat the remaining 1 teaspoon oil. Carefully break the eggs, one at a time, into the skillet, and sprinkle with pepper. Cook about 2 minutes, or until the white is partly set. Carefully flip the eggs and cook 2 minutes longer.

3. Remove the eggs from the skillet and top 4 muffin halves. Return the skillet to the stove, add the bacon, and cook 30 seconds per side. Top eggs with the bacon and spinach, and spread the cut side of the top halves of the muffins with the remaining pesto and set over the spinach.

■ **Eat One Serving:**

299

CALORIES,
20 g protein, 29 g carbohydrates, 16 g fat, 3.2 g saturated fat, 230 mg cholesterol, 825 mg sodium*, 10 g fiber

MAKE IT A FLAT BELLY DIET MEAL:
Add 1 medium banana (105).

■ **Total Meal:**

404

CALORIES

* Limit saturated fat to no more than 10% of total calories—about 20 grams for most men—and sodium intake to no more than 2,300 milligrams.

Spicy Chicken Cheese Steak with Caramelized Onions and Peppers

Preparation time: 10 minutes / Cooking time: 16 minutes / Makes 4 servings

MUFA: ¼ cup olive oil

12 ounces boneless skinless chicken breast halves, thinly sliced

1 onion, thinly sliced

1 green bell pepper, thinly sliced

1 teaspoon dried oregano

¼ teaspoon crushed red-pepper flakes

3 cloves garlic, thinly sliced

2 teaspoons Worcestershire sauce

¼ teaspoon salt

2 ounces shredded 50% reduced-fat sharp Cheddar cheese

1 (8-ounce) French baguette, split lengthwise

1. Heat 2 tablespoons oil in a large nonstick skillet over medium-high heat. Add the chicken and cook, stirring occasionally, 4 to 5 minutes, or until cooked through. Transfer to a plate and reserve. Return the skillet to the stove and heat the remaining 2 tablespoons oil. Add the onion, bell pepper, oregano, and red-pepper flakes. Cook, stirring occasionally, 8 to 9 minutes, or until the onions are golden. Stir in the garlic and cook 1 minute, or until starting to brown. Add the chicken, Worcestershire sauce, and salt. Cook 1 minute, or until hot. Remove from the heat and add in the cheese, stirring until melted.

2. Top the baguette with the chicken mixture. Cut into 4 portions and serve.

■ **Eat One Serving:**

419

CALORIES,
27 g protein, 37 g carbohydrates, 18 g fat, 3.9 g saturated fat, 47 mg cholesterol, 473 mg sodium, 1 g fiber

A SINGLE SERVING OF THIS RECIPE COUNTS AS A FLAT BELLY DIET MEAL WITHOUT ANY ADD-ONS!

Chicken Muffulettas

Preparation time: 15 minutes / Makes 4 servings

**MUFA: 40
Manzanilla
olives, chopped**

½ roasted red-
   pepper,
   chopped
½ clove garlic,
   minced
1 tablespoon red
   wine vinegar
1 tablespoon
   extra-virgin
   olive oil
4 (1½-ounce)
   Portuguese
   rolls, split
4 slices (3 ounces)
   reduced-fat
   provolone
   cheese
8 ounces cooked
   boneless
   skinless chicken
   breast, sliced

1. Combine the olives, roasted pepper, garlic, vinegar, and oil in a bowl and mix well.

2. Arrange the bottom half of each roll on a work surface. Spread half the olive mixture over each. Top with 1 slice of provolone and 2 ounces of sliced chicken. Spoon the remaining olive mixture over the chicken and brush any remaining liquid on the cut side of the top half of each roll. Replace the top half of the rolls, pressing down slightly. Wrap each tightly in plastic wrap and refrigerate at least 1 hour or up to overnight before serving.

■ **Eat One Serving:**

382

CALORIES,
27 g protein, 26 g carbohydrates, 18 g fat, 3.8 g saturated fat, 60 mg cholesterol, 1,235 mg sodium*, 3 g fiber

A SINGLE SERVING OF THIS RECIPE COUNTS AS A FLAT BELLY DIET MEAL WITHOUT ANY ADD-ONS!

* Limit saturated fat to no more than 10% of total calories—about 20 grams for most men— and sodium intake to no more than 2,300 milligrams.

Peanut-Studded Texas Barbecue–Style Chicken Sloppy Joes

Preparation time: 10 minutes / Cooking time: 14 minutes / Makes 4 servings

1 tablespoon olive oil

1 small onion, chopped

½ green bell pepper, chopped

½ jalapeño pepper, finely chopped

2 cloves garlic, minced

1 teaspoon chili powder

1 teaspoon ground cumin

1 teaspoon dried oregano

12 ounces ground chicken breast

½ cup ketchup

1 tablespoon packed dark brown sugar

MUFA: ½ cup unsalted dry-roasted peanuts, coarsely chopped

4 hamburger rolls

1. Heat the oil in a large nonstick skillet over medium-high heat. Add the onion, bell pepper, and jalapeño. Cook, stirring occasionally, 4 to 5 minutes, or until softened.

2. Add the garlic and cook 1 minute. Stir in the chili powder, cumin, and oregano. Cook 15 seconds, until fragrant.

3. Add the chicken and cook, breaking into smaller pieces with a wooden spoon, 3 to 4 minutes, or until no longer pink.

4. Stir in the ketchup and sugar and cook 2 to 3 minutes, until thickened. Stir in the peanuts and cook 1 minute longer.

5. Divide the mixture among the hamburger rolls and serve.

■ **Eat One Serving:**

391

CALORIES,
28 g protein, 40 g carbohydrates, 16 g fat, 2.8 g saturated fat, 49 mg cholesterol, 662 mg sodium*, 3 g fiber

A SINGLE SERVING OF THIS RECIPE COUNTS AS A FLAT BELLY DIET MEAL WITHOUT ANY ADD-ONS!

* Limit saturated fat to no more than 10% of total calories—about 20 grams for most men—and sodium intake to no more than 2,300 milligrams.

Romaine Roast Beef Wraps with Horseradish Cream

Preparation time: 10 minutes / Makes 4 servings

MUFA: ¼ cup olive oil mayonnaise

- 2 teaspoons drained prepared horseradish
- 4 large romaine lettuce leaves, woody vein trimmed at bottom
- ½ golden delicious apple, cut into 16 slices
- 4 ounces reduced-fat thin-sliced Swiss cheese
- 12 ounces deli-sliced roast beef
- 1 tomato, cut into 8 slices

1. Combine the mayonnaise and horseradish in a bowl.

2. Arrange the lettuce leaves on a work surface. Spread the center of each with one-quarter of the mayonnaise mixture. Top each with 4 apple slices, 1 slice of cheese, one-quarter of the roast beef, and 2 tomato slices. Fold each leaf around the filling and serve.

■ **Eat One Serving:**

287

CALORIES,

31 g protein, 6 g carbohydrates, 15 g fat, 5.4 g saturated fat*, 64 mg cholesterol, 231 mg sodium, 1 g fiber

MAKE IT A FLAT BELLY DIET MEAL:

Serve with 4 ounces cooked new potatoes (73) and 1 peach (59).

■ **Total Meal:**

419

CALORIES

* Limit saturated fat to no more than 10% of total calories—about 20 grams for most men—and sodium intake to no more than 2,300 milligrams.

Lamb Souvlaki Pita
with Pine Nut Tzatziki

Preparation time: 10 minutes / Cooking time: 8 minutes / Makes 4 servings

12 ounces lean leg
of lamb,
trimmed, cut
into 16 cubes
4 cloves garlic,
minced
2 tablespoons
lemon juice
1 teaspoon dried
oregano

**MUFA: ½ cup
pine nuts, toasted**

½ cup fat-free
Greek-style
plain yogurt
½ cucumber,
peeled, seeded,
grated, excess
liquid squeezed
out
¼ teaspoon salt
4 whole wheat or
multigrain pitas,
top ⅓ cut off
1 cup shredded
romaine lettuce
1 tomato, cut into
8 slices
¼ red onion,
thinly sliced

1. Combine the lamb, 3 cloves
garlic, lemon juice, and oregano in
a bowl. Refrigerate 30 minutes.

2. Meanwhile, combine the pine
nuts, yogurt, cucumber, remaining
1 clove garlic, and ⅛ teaspoon salt
in a bowl.

3. Preheat the broiler. Coat a
broiler pan with cooking spray.

4. Remove the lamb cubes from
the bowl and thread onto 4
skewers. Sprinkle with remaining
⅛ teaspoon salt. Set on the broiler
pan. Broil lamb 5″ from the heat,
turning often, 6 to 8 minutes.
Remove the lamb from the
skewers. Fill each pita with ¼ cup
lettuce, 4 lamb cubes, 2 tomato
slices, one-quarter of the red
onion, and one-quarter of the
pine nut mixture.

■ **Eat One Serving:**

405

CALORIES,
29 g protein, 35 g
carbohydrates, 18 g
fat, 2.6 g saturated
fat, 55 mg
cholesterol, 539 mg
sodium, 6 g fiber

**A SINGLE SERVING
OF THIS RECIPE
COUNTS AS A
FLAT BELLY DIET
MEAL WITHOUT
ANY ADD-ONS!**

Spice-Rubbed Fresh Tuna Tacos with Cilantro-Avocado-Lime Cream

Preparation time: 10 minutes / Cooking time: 6 minutes / Makes 4 servings

1 teaspoon ground cumin
1 teaspoon chili powder
½ teaspoon garlic powder
½ teaspoon salt
¼ teaspoon black pepper
4 (4-ounce) tuna steaks

MUFA: 1 Hass avocado

¼ cup loosely packed fresh cilantro leaves
¼ cup light sour cream
1 tablespoon lime juice
8 corn tortillas
½ white onion, thinly sliced

1. Combine the cumin, chili powder, garlic powder, ¼ teaspoon salt, and pepper in a bowl. Rub over the tuna steaks and let stand for 10 minutes.

2. Meanwhile, combine the avocado, cilantro, sour cream, lime juice, and remaining ¼ teaspoon salt in a food processor and puree.

3. Preheat a ridged grill pan that has been coated with cooking spray. Add the tuna and cook 2 to 3 minutes per side, or until well marked and cooked through. Transfer to a cutting board. Thinly slice the tuna.

4. Heat tortillas over a gas burner, turning occasionally, about 1 minute, or place the tortillas between clean paper towels and microwave on high for 15 to 20 seconds to warm. Fill the tortillas with sliced tuna and onion and top with the cilantro-avocado cream.

■ **Eat One Serving:**

312

CALORIES,
31 g protein, 29 g carbohydrates, 9 g fat, 1.9 g saturated fat, 56 mg cholesterol, 374 mg sodium, 6 g fiber

MAKE IT A FLAT BELLY DIET MEAL:
Serve with ½ cup mango (60).

■ **Total Meal:**

372

CALORIES

Grilled Catfish Po' Boy Topped with Peanut Slaw

Preparation time: 10 minutes / Cooking time: 12 minutes / Makes 4 servings

2 cups classic coleslaw mix

MUFA: ½ cup unsalted dry-roasted peanuts

2 tablespoons cider vinegar

2 teaspoons sugar

¼ teaspoon salt

2 (6-ounce) catfish fillets

1 teaspoon Cajun seasoning

1 (8-ounce) French baguette, split lengthwise

1 plum tomato, cut into 8 slices

1. Combine the coleslaw mix, peanuts, vinegar, sugar, and salt in a bowl. Let stand 30 minutes.

2. Preheat a grill pan that has been coated with cooking spray.

3. Sprinkle the catfish with Cajun seasoning and add to the grill pan. Cook 5 to 6 minutes per side, or until the fish flakes easily with a fork.

4. Set the bottom half of the baguette on a work surface. Top with the tomato slices, catfish fillets, and coleslaw. Replace the top half of the baguette and cut into 4 portions. Serve immediately.

■ **Eat One Serving:**

392

CALORIES,
23 g protein, 39 g carbohydrates, 16 g fat, 2.8 g saturated fat, 40 mg cholesterol, 631 mg sodium*, 2 g fiber

A SINGLE SERVING OF THIS RECIPE COUNTS AS A FLAT BELLY DIET MEAL WITHOUT ANY ADD-ONS!

* Limit saturated fat to no more than 10% of total calories—about 20 grams for most men—and sodium intake to no more than 2,300 milligrams.

Shrimp, Mushroom, and Onion Quesadillas

Preparation time: 10 minutes / Cooking time: 16 minutes / Makes 4 servings

MUFA: ¼ cup olive oil

12 ounces peeled and deveined medium shrimp
¾ teaspoon chili powder
¼ teaspoon salt
1 onion, thinly sliced
1 teaspoon dried oregano
1 (8-ounce) package sliced mushrooms
2 cloves garlic, minced
4 (7") flour tortillas
2 ounces shredded 50% reduced-fat Cheddar cheese

1. Heat 1 tablespoon oil in a large nonstick skillet over medium-high heat. Sprinkle the shrimp with chili powder and ⅛ teaspoon salt. Add to the skillet and cook 2 to 3 minutes per side or until opaque. Transfer to a plate and reserve. Add the remaining 3 tablespoons oil to the skillet and add the onions and oregano. Cook, stirring occasionally, 4 minutes, or until the onions are softened. Add the mushrooms and remaining ⅛ teaspoon salt. Cook, stirring occasionally, 5 to 6 minutes, or until the mushrooms begin to brown. Stir in the garlic and cook 2 minutes. Transfer to a bowl.

2. Arrange the tortillas on a work surface. Sprinkle with cheese. Top the bottom half of each with one-quarter of the onion mixture. Top with the shrimp, then fold the tortilla over to form a semicircle.

3. Heat the skillet over medium heat until hot. Add 2 quesadillas and cook 3 to 4 minutes per side until lightly browned and the filling is hot. Transfer to a cutting board and repeat with the remaining quesadillas. Cut each into 2 wedges and serve.

■ **Eat One Serving:**

401

CALORIES,

27 g protein, 27 g carbohydrates, 22 g fat, 4.7 g saturated fat*, 129 mg cholesterol, 672 mg sodium*, 1 g fiber

A SINGLE SERVING OF THIS RECIPE COUNTS AS A FLAT BELLY DIET MEAL WITHOUT ANY ADD-ONS!

* Limit saturated fat to no more than 10% of total calories—about 20 grams for most men— and sodium intake to no more than 2,300 milligrams.

Chicken Caesar Salad

Preparation time: 15 minutes / Makes 4 servings

MUFA: ¼ cup canola oil mayonnaise

3 tablespoons grated Parmesan cheese

2 tablespoons lemon juice

½ teaspoon anchovy paste

½ clove garlic, minced

½ teaspoon Worcestershire sauce

⅛ teaspoon black pepper

6 cups torn romaine lettuce

2 cups cubed cooked boneless skinless chicken breast

24 fat-free croutons

1. Combine the mayonnaise, Parmesan, lemon juice, anchovy paste, garlic, Worcestershire sauce, and pepper in a bowl. Mix well.

2. Combine the lettuce, chicken, and croutons in a separate bowl. Pour in the mayonnaise mixture and toss well to coat. Divide among 4 bowls and serve.

■ **Eat One Serving:**

305

CALORIES,

25 g protein, 8 g carbohydrates, 18 g fat, 2.1 g saturated fat, 67 mg cholesterol, 310 mg sodium, 2 g fiber

MAKE IT A FLAT BELLY DIET MEAL:

Serve with ½ cup of low-fat vanilla yogurt (104).

■ **Total Meal:**

409

CALORIES

Grilled Chicken and Cherry Tomato Pasta Salad

Preparation time: 15 minutes / Cooking time: 12 minutes / Makes 4 servings

4 ounces rotini
pasta

2 cups broccoli
florets

4 (4-ounce)
boneless
skinless chicken
breast halves

**MUFA: 2
teaspoons olive
oil + ¼ cup extra-
virgin olive oil**

½ teaspoon salt

¼ teaspoon black
pepper

1 cup grape
tomatoes,
halved

¼ red onion,
thinly sliced

¼ cup thinly sliced
fresh basil

2 tablespoons
grated Romano
cheese

2 tablespoons
lemon juice

1. Bring a large pot of lightly salted water to a boil. Add the pasta and cook according to package directions. Add the broccoli during the last 3 minutes of cooking. Drain, rinse under cold water, and drain well again. Transfer to a bowl.

2. Heat a grill pan coated with cooking spray over medium-high heat. Brush the chicken with 2 teaspoons oil, ¼ teaspoon salt, and ⅛ teaspoon pepper. Add to the grill pan and cook 6 to 7 minutes per side, or until a thermometer inserted into the thickest portion registers 165°F. Transfer to a cutting board and cool 5 minutes. Cut into ½" cubes and add to the bowl with the pasta. Stir in the ¼ cup oil, ¼ teaspoon salt, ⅛ teaspoon pepper, tomatoes, onion, basil, Romano, and lemon juice. Toss well.

3. Divide among 4 serving bowls.

■ **Eat One Serving:**

408

CALORIES,
30 g protein, 26 g
carbohydrates, 21 g
fat, 3.9 g saturated
fat, 66 mg
cholesterol, 422 mg
sodium, 3 g fiber

**A SINGLE SERVING
OF THIS RECIPE
COUNTS AS A
FLAT BELLY DIET
MEAL WITHOUT
ANY ADD-ONS!**

Flank Steak Chopped Steakhouse Salad

Preparation time: 15 minutes / Cooking time: 12 minutes / Makes 4 servings

1 pound lean
  flank steak,
  trimmed
³⁄₈ teaspoon salt
³⁄₈ teaspoon black
  pepper
2 romaine lettuce
  hearts, chopped,
  about 6 cups
4 plum tomatoes,
  seeded and
  chopped
1 cucumber,
  peeled, seeded,
  and chopped
1 large carrot,
  chopped
½ medium red
  onion, finely
  chopped
⅓ cup reduced-fat
  crumbled blue
  cheese

MUFA: ¼ **cup**
canola oil
mayonnaise

3 tablespoons
  light sour cream
1 tablespoon white
  wine vinegar
½ teaspoon
  Worcestershire
  sauce

1. Prepare the grill for medium-high heat.

2. Sprinkle the flank steak with ¼ teaspoon salt and ¼ teaspoon pepper. Place the steak on a grill rack coated with cooking spray. Grill 5 to 6 minutes per side, or until desired doneness. Transfer to a cutting board and let rest 10 minutes before thinly slicing.

3. Meanwhile, combine the romaine, tomatoes, cucumber, carrot, and onion in a large bowl. Combine the blue cheese, mayonnaise, sour cream, vinegar, Worcestershire sauce, and the remaining ¼ teaspoon of pepper in a separate bowl. Add the cheese mixture to the romaine mixture and toss well to coat. Divide among 4 serving bowls and top each with ¼ of the sliced steak.

■ **Eat One Serving:**

343

CALORIES,
29 g protein, 10 g carbohydrates, 20 g fat, 4.6 g saturated fat*, 51 mg cholesterol, 531 mg sodium, 3 g fiber

MAKE IT A FLAT BELLY DIET MEAL:
Serve with 1 medium tangerine (47).

■ **Total Meal:**

390

CALORIES

* Limit saturated fat to no more than 10% of total calories—about 20 grams for most men—and sodium intake to no more than 2,300 milligrams.

Spaghetti Fra Diavolo with Chicken Meatballs

Preparation time: 20 minutes / Cooking time: 25 minutes / Makes 4 servings

12 ounces ground chicken or turkey breast
1 egg white
¼ cup Italian seasoned bread crumbs
½ teaspoon salt
⅛ teaspoon black pepper

MUFA: ¼ cup extra-virgin olive oil

3 cloves garlic, minced
1 teaspoon dried oregano
¼ teaspoon crushed red-pepper flakes
1 (14.5-ounce) can crushed tomatoes
6 ounces spaghetti

1. Combine the ground chicken, egg white, bread crumbs, ¼ teaspoon salt, and pepper in a bowl. With lightly moistened hands, form the mixture into 12 (1½″) balls. Heat 1 tablespoon oil in a large nonstick skillet over medium-high heat. Add the meatballs and cook, turning occasionally, 5 to 6 minutes, or until browned. Transfer to a plate and reserve.

2. Bring a large pot of lightly salted water to a boil.

3. Return the skillet to the stove and heat the remaining 3 tablespoons oil over medium-high heat. Add the garlic, oregano, and red-pepper flakes. Cook 30 seconds. Stir in the tomatoes and bring to a boil, then reduce the heat to medium-low, cover, and simmer 6 to 7 minutes, until starting to thicken. Add the remaining ¼ teaspoon of salt and the meatballs and simmer 8 to 9 minutes longer, or until the meatballs are cooked through.

4. Meanwhile, add the spaghetti to the boiling water and cook according to package directions, then drain. Divide the spaghetti among 4 bowls, and top each with sauce and 3 meatballs.

■ **Eat One Serving:**

429

CALORIES,
28 g protein, 45 g carbohydrates, 16 g fat, 2.1 g saturated fat, 49 mg cholesterol, 607 mg sodium*, 4 g fiber

A SINGLE SERVING OF THIS RECIPE COUNTS AS A FLAT BELLY DIET MEAL WITHOUT ANY ADD-ONS!

* Limit saturated fat to no more than 10% of total calories—about 20 grams for most men—and sodium intake to no more than 2,300 milligrams.

Rotini with Turkey Sausage, Garlic, and Oil

Preparation time: 5 minutes / Cooking time: 20 minutes / Makes 4 servings

6 ounces rotini pasta

MUFA: ¼ cup extra-virgin olive oil

8 ounces Italian-style turkey sausage, removed from casings

1 teaspoon dried oregano

⅛ teaspoon crushed red-pepper flakes

1 pint grape tomatoes

8 cloves garlic, thinly sliced

¼ teaspoon salt

3 tablespoons chopped fresh parsley

1. Bring a large pot of lightly salted water to a boil. Add the pasta and cook according to package directions, then drain.

2. Meanwhile, heat the oil in a large nonstick skillet over medium-high heat. Add the sausage, oregano, and red-pepper flakes. Cook, breaking sausage into smaller pieces with a wooden spoon, 5 to 6 minutes, or until starting to brown. Stir in the tomatoes and garlic. Cook, stirring occasionally, 2½ to 3 minutes, or until tomatoes wilt and garlic is lightly browned. Add the pasta and salt. Toss about 30 seconds, until hot. Remove from the heat and stir in the parsley. Serve immediately.

■ Eat One Serving:

400

CALORIES,

16 g protein, 38 g carbohydrates, 21 g fat, 2.2 g saturated fat, 34 mg cholesterol, 518 mg sodium, 3 g fiber

A SINGLE SERVING OF THIS RECIPE COUNTS AS A FLAT BELLY DIET MEAL WITHOUT ANY ADD-ONS!

Penne Bolognese

Preparation time: 5 minutes / Cooking time: 20 minutes / Makes 4 servings

6 ounces penne
pasta

**MUFA: ¼ cup
extra-virgin olive
oil**

8 ounces extra-
lean ground
round beef

1 teaspoon dried
basil

1 medium onion,
chopped

1 medium carrot,
finely chopped

3 cloves garlic,
minced

1 (14.5-ounce)
can fire-roasted
diced tomatoes

3 tablespoons
tomato paste

¼ cup grated
Parmesan
cheese

¼ teaspoon black
pepper

1. Bring a large pot of lightly
salted water to a boil. Add the
pasta and cook according to
package directions, then drain.

2. Heat the oil in a large nonstick
skillet over medium-high heat.
Add the beef and basil. Cook,
breaking the beef into smaller
pieces with a wooden spoon, 4 to
5 minutes, or until starting to
brown. Stir in the onion, carrot,
and garlic, and cook 3 to 4
minutes, until the beef is browned
and the vegetables are slightly
softened. Add the tomatoes and
tomato paste and bring to a boil.
Reduce the heat to medium and
simmer 10 minutes. Remove from
the heat, stir in the Parmesan and
pepper, and serve over the pasta.

■ Eat One Serving:

422

CALORIES,
21 g protein, 44 g
carbohydrates, 18 g
fat, 3.8 g saturated
fat, 34 mg
cholesterol, 585 mg
sodium, 4 g fiber

**A SINGLE SERVING
OF THIS RECIPE
COUNTS AS A
FLAT BELLY DIET
MEAL WITHOUT
ANY ADD-ONS!**

Spicy Linguine with Bacon and White Clam Sauce

Preparation time: 10 minutes / Cooking time: 10–12 minutes / Makes 4 servings

8 ounces linguine

MUFA: ¼ cup extra-virgin olive oil

3 slices bacon, chopped

¼ – ½ teaspoon crushed red-pepper flakes

1 onion, chopped

1 teaspoon dried oregano

4 cloves garlic, minced

2 (6½-ounce) cans chopped clams, drained

1 (8-ounce) bottle clam juice

¼ teaspoon salt

¼ cup chopped fresh parsley

1. Bring a large pot of lightly salted water to a boil. Add the linguine and cook according to package directions, then drain.

2. Meanwhile, heat the oil in a large nonstick skillet over medium-high heat. Add the bacon and red-pepper flakes. Cook, stirring occasionally, until just starting to brown. Stir in the onion and oregano and cook 2 to 3 minutes, until starting to soften. Add the garlic and cook 1 to 2 minutes. Stir in the clams, clam juice, and salt. Bring to a boil and cook 2 to 4 minutes, until slightly reduced. Stir in the linguine and parsley. Toss 1 minute, or until hot.

■ **Eat One Serving:**

437

CALORIES,
21 g protein, 48 g carbohydrates, 18 g fat, 2.9 g saturated fat, 34 mg cholesterol, 429 mg sodium, 3 g fiber

A SINGLE SERVING OF THIS RECIPE COUNTS AS A FLAT BELLY DIET MEAL WITHOUT ANY ADD-ONS!

PASTA & PIZZA

Orecchiette with Garlic and Pesto

Preparation time: 5 minutes / Cooking time: 12 minutes / Makes 4 servings

8 ounces orecchiette pasta
1 tablespoon extra-virgin olive oil
1 medium onion, thinly sliced
5 cloves garlic, thinly sliced

MUFA: ¼ cup pesto

¼ teaspoon salt
¼ teaspoon black pepper
8 teaspoons grated Romano cheese

1. Bring a large pot of lightly salted water to a boil. Add the pasta and cook according to package directions. Drain and transfer to a bowl.

2. Heat the oil in a medium nonstick skillet over medium-high heat. Add the onions and cook 5 to 6 minutes, stirring occasionally, until starting to brown. Stir in the garlic and cook about 2 minutes, until lightly browned. Add to the pasta. Stir in the pesto, salt, and pepper. Divide among 4 plates and sprinkle each with 2 teaspoons Romano.

■ **Eat One Serving:**

345

CALORIES,
12 g protein, 46 g carbohydrates, 13 g fat, 3.3 g saturated fat, 8 mg cholesterol, 342 mg sodium, 3 g fiber

MAKE IT A FLAT BELLY DIET MEAL:

Serve with 1 cup of steamed or roasted Brussels sprouts (56).

■ **Total Meal:**

401

CALORIES

Black and Red Bean Chili with Wagon Wheels

Preparation time: 10 minutes / Cooking time: 30 minutes / Makes 4 servings

4 ounces wagon
   wheel pasta

MUFA: ¼ **cup
olive oil**

2 onions, chopped
1 green bell
   pepper, chopped
1 red bell pepper,
   chopped
4 cloves garlic,
   minced
1 tablespoon chili
   powder
1 teaspoon
   ground cumin
1 teaspoon dried
   oregano
1 (15-ounce) can
   no-salt-added
   black beans,
   drained and
   rinsed
1 (15-ounce) can
   no-salt-added
   red kidney
   beans, drained
   and rinsed
1 (15-ounce) can
   fire-roasted
   diced tomatoes
½ cup water
½ ounce semisweet
   chocolate
¼ teaspoon salt

1. Bring a pot of lightly salted water to a boil. Add the pasta and cook according to package directions, then drain.

2. Meanwhile, heat the oil in a Dutch oven over medium-high heat. Add the onions, bell peppers, and garlic. Cook 6 to 7 minutes, stirring occasionally, until crisp-tender. Stir in the chili powder, cumin, and oregano and cook 1 minute. Add the black beans, kidney beans, tomatoes, and water. Bring to a boil, reduce heat to medium-low, cover, and simmer 30 minutes. Remove from the heat and add the chocolate and salt, stirring until the chocolate has melted. Serve over the pasta.

■ **Eat One Serving:**

426

CALORIES,
14 g protein, 61 g carbohydrates, 16 g fat, 2.7 g saturated fat, 0 mg cholesterol, 516 mg sodium, 14 g fiber

A SINGLE SERVING OF THIS RECIPE COUNTS AS A FLAT BELLY DIET MEAL WITHOUT ANY ADD-ONS!

Mexican Seafood Pizza

Preparation time: 10 minutes / Cooking time: 20 minutes / Makes 4 servings

2 (10") flour
tortillas
2 teaspoons olive
oil
6 ounces peeled
and deveined
medium shrimp
6 ounces bay
scallops
2/3 cup prepared
mild salsa

**MUFA: 1 Hass
avocado, peeled,
pitted, and thinly
sliced**

4 ounces shredded
reduced-fat
Mexican blend
cheese
2 tablespoons
chopped fresh
cilantro

1. Preheat the oven to 425°F.
Coat 2 baking sheets with
cooking spray.

2. Set 1 tortilla on each baking
sheet and lightly coat with
cooking spray. Bake 6 to 7
minutes, until lightly browned
and crisp. Remove from the oven
and cool.

3. Meanwhile, heat the oil in a
large nonstick skillet over
medium-high heat. Add the
shrimp and scallops and cook
2 to 3 minutes per side. Transfer
to a plate.

4. Spread each tortilla with
1/3 cup salsa, leaving a 3/4" border
around the edge of each. Top
each with avocado slices, cheese,
shrimp, and scallops. Bake 6 to
7 minutes, until the cheese melts.
Remove from the oven, sprinkle
with cilantro, and cut each into
4 wedges.

■ **Eat One Serving:**

363

CALORIES,

27 g protein, 26 g
carbohydrates, 17 g
fat, 4.9 g saturated
fat*, 99 mg
cholesterol, 712 mg
sodium*, 3 g fiber

**A SINGLE SERVING
OF THIS RECIPE
COUNTS AS A
FLAT BELLY DIET
MEAL WITHOUT
ANY ADD-ONS!**

* Limit saturated fat to no
more than 10% of total
calories—about 20
grams for most men—
and sodium intake to no
more than 2,300
milligrams.

Cashew Beef with Broccoli and Snow Peas

Preparation time: 10 minutes / Cooking time: 8 minutes / Makes 4 servings

1 pound extra-lean top round steak, thinly sliced

3 tablespoons dry sherry

2 tablespoons low-sodium soy sauce

1 tablespoon honey

2 teaspoons black bean sauce

1 tablespoon Asian sesame oil

1 onion, chopped

1 tablespoon grated fresh ginger

3 cups broccoli florets

1/3 cup water

4 ounces snow peas

1 carrot, sliced

MUFA: 1/2 cup unsalted roasted cashews

1. Combine the steak, 1 tablespoon sherry, and 1 tablespoon soy sauce in a bowl. Combine the remaining 2 tablespoons sherry, 1 tablespoon soy sauce, honey, and black bean sauce in a separate bowl.

2. Heat 1 teaspoon oil in a large nonstick skillet over medium-high heat until it just begins to smoke. Add the steak and cook, stirring occasionally, for 2 minutes, or until it is no longer pink. Transfer to a plate and reserve. Return the skillet to heat and add the remaining 2 teaspoons oil. Stir in the onion and cook 1 minute. Add the ginger and cook, stirring, 15 seconds, until fragrant. Add the broccoli and water. Cook 2 minutes, stirring often, until broccoli is bright green. Stir in the snow peas, carrot, and cashews. Cook 2 minutes, stirring often. Stir in the beef and sherry mixture. Cook about 1 minute, until hot and the vegetables are crisp-tender.

■ **Eat One Serving:**

314

CALORIES,
30 g protein, 20 g carbohydrates, 15 g fat, 3.7 g saturated fat, 50 mg cholesterol, 407 mg sodium, 4 g fiber

MAKE IT A FLAT BELLY DIET MEAL:
Serve with 1 cup pineapple chunks (108).

■ **Total Meal:**

422

CALORIES

Italian Sausage Skillet with Caramelized Onions, Tomatoes, and Peppers

Preparation time: 15 minutes / Cooking time: 40 minutes / Makes 4 servings

3 sweet Italian sausages (12 ounces)
½ cup water

MUFA: ¼ cup extra-virgin olive oil

1 large onion, sliced
1 teaspoon sugar
1 teaspoon dried basil
1 teaspoon dried oregano
1 red bell pepper, sliced
1 green bell pepper, sliced
3 cloves garlic, sliced
3 plum tomatoes, cut into 16 pieces each
1 tablespoon balsamic vinegar
⅛ teaspoon salt
¼ teaspoon black pepper

1. Combine the sausage with the water in a small nonstick skillet over medium-high heat. Cook 15 to 17 minutes, turning sausage occasionally, until the water is evaporated and the sausage is browned and cooked through. Transfer to a cutting board. Cool 5 minutes and cut into ½"-thick slices.

2. Heat the oil in a large nonstick skillet over medium-high heat. Add the onion, sugar, basil, and oregano. Cook, stirring occasionally, for 12 to 14 minutes, or until golden. Stir in the bell peppers and cook 3 to 4 minutes, until crisp-tender. Add the garlic and cook 1 minute. Add the tomatoes and cook 3 to 4 minutes, until wilted. Stir in the sausage, vinegar, salt, and pepper. Cook about 1 minute, until hot.

Eat One Serving:

304

CALORIES,
15 g protein, 13 g carbohydrates, 22 g fat, 4.8 g saturated fat*, 26 mg cholesterol, 565 mg sodium, 3 g fiber

MAKE IT A FLAT BELLY DIET MEAL:
Serve with 1 slice (1 ounce) whole grain French bread (90).

Total Meal:

394

CALORIES

* Limit saturated fat to no more than 10% of total calories—about 20 grams for most men—and sodium intake to no more than 2,300 milligrams.

Pulled Pork Sliders with Creamy Coleslaw

Preparation time: 10 minutes / Cooking time: 65 minutes / Makes 4 servings

12 ounces lean pork tenderloin, trimmed, cut into 8 pieces

½ cup barbecue sauce

3 tablespoons cider vinegar

4 cups classic coleslaw mix

MUFA: ¼ cup canola oil mayonnaise

2 teaspoons sugar

¼ teaspoon black pepper

8 (⅓-ounce) whole wheat potato rolls

1. Combine the pork, barbecue sauce, and 2 tablespoons vinegar in a medium saucepan over medium-high heat. Bring to a boil, reduce heat to medium-low, cover and simmer, stirring occasionally, for 60 to 65 minutes, until very tender. Remove from the heat and shred with two forks.

2. Meanwhile, combine the remaining 1 tablespoon vinegar, coleslaw mix, mayonnaise, sugar, and pepper in a bowl and toss well.

3. Fill the rolls with pork and serve with coleslaw.

■ **Eat One Serving:**

437

CALORIES,
32 g protein, 50 g carbohydrates, 15 g fat, 1 g saturated fat, 60 mg cholesterol, 792 mg sodium*, 9 g fiber

A SINGLE SERVING OF THIS RECIPE COUNTS AS A FLAT BELLY DIET MEAL WITHOUT ANY ADD-ONS!

* Limit saturated fat to no more than 10% of total calories—about 20 grams for most men— and sodium intake to no more than 2,300 milligrams.

Pan-Seared Salmon Fillet with Tomato, Basil, and Kalamata Olives

Preparation time: 15 minutes / Cooking time: 12 minutes / Makes 4 servings

MUFA: 40 Kalamata olives, finely chopped

- 2 cups grape tomatoes, quartered
- 3 tablespoons chopped fresh basil
- 2 teaspoons lemon juice
- 2 teaspoons extra-virgin olive oil
- 1 teaspoon drained capers, minced
- 1 clove garlic, minced
- 4 (4-ounce) skinless salmon fillets
- $\frac{1}{8}$ teaspoon salt
- $\frac{1}{4}$ teaspoon black pepper

1. Combine the olives, tomatoes, basil, lemon juice, oil, capers, and garlic in a bowl. Mix well.

2. Heat a large nonstick skillet over medium-high heat. Sprinkle the salmon with salt and pepper and add to the skillet. Cook 10 to 12 minutes, turning once, until fish flakes easily with a fork. Serve topped with the olive mixture.

■ Eat One Serving:

350

CALORIES,
24 g protein, 7 g carbohydrates, 25 g fat, 4 g saturated fat*, 67 mg cholesterol, 703 mg sodium*, 1 g fiber

MAKE IT A FLAT BELLY DIET MEAL:
Serve with $\frac{1}{2}$ cup of cooked peas (67).

■ Total Meal:

417

CALORIES

* Limit saturated fat to no more than 10% of total calories—about 20 grams for most men— and sodium intake to no more than 2,300 milligrams.

Hoisin-Peanut Stir-Fry with Tofu, Mushrooms, and Peas

Preparation time: 5 minutes / Cooking time: 19 minutes / Makes 4 servings

4 teaspoons canola oil

1 (14-ounce) package extra-firm light tofu, drained, pressed, cut into ½" pieces

1 onion, chopped

1 (8-ounce) package sliced mushrooms

3 cloves garlic, minced

1 tablespoon grated fresh ginger

½ cup frozen peas

MUFA: ½ cup dry-roasted unsalted peanuts

⅓ cup hoisin sauce

1 tablespoon seasoned rice vinegar

3 green onions, chopped

2 cups hot cooked brown rice

1. Heat 2 teaspoons oil in a large nonstick skillet over medium-high heat. Add the tofu and cook 8 to 10 minutes, turning occasionally, until lightly browned. Transfer to a plate and reserve.

2. Return the skillet to the stove and heat the remaining 2 teaspoons oil. Stir in the onion and cook 1 minute. Add the mushrooms and cook 5 to 6 minutes, stirring occasionally, until lightly browned. Stir in the garlic and ginger and cook 30 seconds, until fragrant. Add the peas and peanuts and cook 1 minute, until the peas are bright green. Add the tofu, hoisin, and vinegar. Cook, stirring, for 1 minute, or until hot.

3. Remove from the heat and stir in the green onions. Serve over rice.

■ **Eat One Serving:**

402

CALORIES,
20 g protein, 46 g carbohydrates, 18 g fat, 1.9 g saturated fat, 1 mg cholesterol, 483 mg sodium, 7 g fiber

A SINGLE SERVING OF THIS RECIPE COUNTS AS A FLAT BELLY DIET MEAL WITHOUT ANY ADD-ONS!

Baked Chicken Nuggets with Chipotle Mayonnaise

Preparation time: 15 minutes / Cooking time: 12 minutes / Makes 4 servings

3 tablespoons all-purpose flour

1 teaspoon paprika

1 teaspoon ground cumin

½ teaspoon garlic powder

½ teaspoon salt

1 egg, lightly beaten

1 tablespoon water

1 cup cornflake crumbs

1 pound boneless skinless chicken breast halves, cut into 24 pieces

MUFA: ¼ cup canola oil mayonnaise

2 teaspoons lime juice

½ chipotle pepper en adobo, minced

1. Preheat the oven to 425°F. Coat a large baking sheet with cooking spray.

2. Combine the flour, paprika, cumin, garlic powder, and salt in a bowl. Place the egg in a separate bowl and mix with the water. Place the cornflake crumbs in a third bowl. Working a few pieces at a time, coat the chicken with the flour mixture, shaking off any excess. Then dip into the egg mixture to coat and dredge in the cornflake crumbs. Place the coated nuggets on the prepared baking sheet and repeat with the remaining chicken.

3. Lightly coat the chicken nuggets with cooking spray. Bake 10 minutes, turn over, and bake 2 to 5 minutes longer, or until crisp and golden.

4. Meanwhile, combine the mayonnaise, lime juice, and chipotle pepper in a small bowl. Serve with the chicken nuggets.

■ **Eat One Serving:**

348

CALORIES,

27 g protein, 25 g carbohydrates, 15 g fat, 1.6 g saturated fat, 121 mg cholesterol, 622 mg sodium*, 1 g fiber

MAKE IT A FLAT BELLY DIET MEAL:

Serve with ½ cup roasted baby potatoes (70).

■ **Total Meal:**

418

CALORIES

* Limit saturated fat to no more than 10% of total calories—about 20 grams for most men—and sodium intake to no more than 2,300 milligrams.

Almond-Crusted Chicken Breasts with Balsamic Drizzle

Preparation time: 10 minutes / Cooking time: 15 minutes / Makes 4 servings

1 large egg

1 tablespoon water

MUFA: ½ cup almonds, finely chopped

¼ cup Italian seasoned bread crumbs

½ teaspoon salt

4 (5-ounce) boneless skinless chicken breast halves

½ cup orange juice

½ cup balsamic vinegar

3 tablespoons honey

1. Preheat the oven to 425°F. Coat a baking sheet with cooking spray.

2. Whisk the egg with the water in a shallow bowl. Combine the almonds, bread crumbs, and salt in another shallow bowl. Dip the chicken into the egg and then the nut mixture. Place on the prepared baking sheet and coat chicken with cooking spray.

3. Bake, turning once, for 15 minutes, or until a thermometer inserted into the thickest portion registers 165°F.

4. Meanwhile, bring the orange juice, vinegar, and honey to a boil in a small saucepan over medium-high heat. Boil 9 to 10 minutes, until reduced by half. Serve over chicken.

■ **Eat One Serving:**

393

CALORIES,

36 g protein, 30 g carbohydrates, 14 g fat, 2 g saturated fat, 131 mg cholesterol, 497 mg sodium, 2 g fiber

A SINGLE SERVING OF THIS RECIPE COUNTS AS A FLAT BELLY DIET MEAL WITHOUT ANY ADD-ONS!

IN THE OVEN

Moroccan-Style Turkey Meatloaf

Preparation time: 10 minutes / Cooking time: 50 minutes / Makes 4 servings

½ cup golden
   raisins
¼ cup orange
   juice
¼ cup water

**MUFA: ½ cup
walnuts**

¼ cup plain dry
   bread crumbs
1 pound lean
   ground turkey
   (7% fat)
1 egg
½ medium onion,
   chopped
¼ cup chopped
   fresh basil
2 tablespoons
   tomato paste
1 teaspoon
   ground cumin
⅛ teaspoon
   ground
   cinnamon
½ teaspoon salt
¼ teaspoon black
   pepper

1. Preheat the oven to 350°F. Coat a large rimmed baking sheet with cooking spray.

2. Combine the raisins, orange juice, and water in a small saucepan over medium-high heat. Bring to a boil, remove from the heat, and let stand 10 minutes, then drain. Meanwhile, combine the walnuts and bread crumbs in the bowl of a food processor. Process until finely ground and transfer to a bowl. Add the drained raisins, turkey, egg, onion, basil, tomato paste, cumin, cinnamon, salt, and pepper. Mix until blended.

3. Shape into a loaf about 7" x 4½" on the prepared baking sheet. Bake 45 to 50 minutes, or until a thermometer inserted into the thickest portion registers 165°F. Let stand 5 minutes before slicing.

■ **Eat One Serving:**

285

CALORIES,
28 g protein, 27 g carbohydrates, 19 g fat, 3.6 g saturated fat, 118 mg cholesterol, 455 mg sodium, 3 g fiber

**MAKE IT A FLAT
BELLY DIET MEAL:**
Serve with 1 medium sweet potato (103).

■ **Total Meal:**

388

CALORIES

Baked Eggplant Pesto Parmesan

Preparation time: 15 minutes / Cooking time: 32 minutes / Makes 4 servings

¼ cup all-purpose flour

1 teaspoon dried basil

¼ teaspoon black pepper

4 large egg whites, lightly beaten

¾ cup plain dry bread crumbs

1 pound eggplant, trimmed, cut into 12 slices

1½ cups low-sodium tomato-basil pasta sauce

MUFA: ¼ cup pesto

1 cup reduced-fat shredded mozzarella cheese

2 tablespoons grated Parmesan cheese

1. Preheat the oven to 450°F. Coat a large baking sheet and an 11" x 7" baking dish with cooking spray.

2. Combine the flour, basil, and pepper in a bowl. Pour the egg whites into a second bowl, and pour the bread crumbs into a third bowl. Working one slice at a time, coat the eggplant with the flour mixture. Then dip into the egg mixture, shaking off the excess, and then dredge both sides in bread crumbs. Place the slice on the prepared baking sheet and repeat with the remaining eggplant slices, being sure to arrange them in a single layer on the baking sheet. Lightly spray the eggplant with cooking spray. Bake 10 minutes, turn the slices, and bake about 10 minutes longer, until golden.

3. Spread ½ cup pasta sauce over the bottom of the prepared baking dish. Arrange 6 eggplant slices in an overlapping pattern. Then spread with the remaining 1 cup pasta sauce. Arrange the remaining eggplant over the sauce. Spread the top slices with pesto, then sprinkle with mozzarella and Parmesan cheeses. Reduce the oven temperature to 350°F. Bake 10 to 12 minutes longer, until the cheese melts.

■ **Eat One Serving:**

392

CALORIES,
22 g protein, 41 g carbohydrates, 16 g fat, 4.2 g saturated fat*, 128 mg cholesterol, 649 mg sodium*, 6 g fiber

A SINGLE SERVING OF THIS RECIPE COUNTS AS A FLAT BELLY DIET MEAL WITHOUT ANY ADD-ONS!

* Limit saturated fat to no more than 10% of total calories—about 20 grams for most men—and sodium intake to less than 2,300 milligrams.

Monterey Jack and Jalapeño Turkey Burgers with Special Sauce

Preparation time: 10 minutes / Cooking time: 7 minutes / Makes 4 servings

MUFA: ¼ cup canola oil mayonnaise

2 tablespoons ketchup

1 teaspoon Dijon mustard

1 pound 99% fat-free lean ground turkey breast

½ small onion, finely chopped

2 ounces reduced-fat Monterey Jack cheese, shredded

4 light multigrain 100-calorie English muffins, split and toasted

4 small romaine lettuce leaves

1 medium tomato, cut into 8 slices

12 pickled jalapeño slices

1. Prepare the grill for direct-heat grilling and coat the grill rack with cooking spray.

2. Combine the mayonnaise, ketchup, and mustard in a bowl and set aside.

3. Combine the turkey, onion, and cheese in a bowl and mix until just blended. Shape into 4 burgers.

4. Set the burgers on the grill rack, directly over the heat source. Cook the burgers, turning once, 7 to 8 minutes, or until well marked and a thermometer inserted into the thickest portion registers 165°F.

5. Place the bottom of each English muffin on 4 plates. Top with 1 lettuce leaf and 2 tomato slices. Place 1 burger on each and top with 3 jalapeño slices, one-quarter of the mayonnaise mixture, and the top of the muffin.

■ **Eat One Serving:**

382

CALORIES,
37 g protein, 29 g carbohydrates, 17 g fat, 2.3 g saturated fat, 60 mg cholesterol, 627 mg sodium*, 9 g fiber

A SINGLE SERVING OF THIS RECIPE COUNTS AS A FLAT BELLY DIET MEAL WITHOUT ANY ADD-ONS!

* Limit saturated fat to no more than 10% of total calories—about 20 grams for most men—and sodium intake to no more than 2,300 milligrams.

Grilled Chicken Breasts with Peanut Barbecue Sauce

Preparation time: 5 minutes / Cooking time: 14 minutes / Makes 4 servings

MUFA: ½ cup unsalted creamy natural peanut butter

- 3 tablespoons ketchup
- 3 tablespoons hoisin sauce
- 1 teaspoon Asian sesame oil
- ¼ cup water
- 4 (4-ounce) boneless skinless chicken breast halves

1. Combine the peanut butter, ketchup, hoisin sauce, sesame oil, and warm water in a bowl. Combine the chicken breasts and ¼ cup peanut butter mixture in a separate bowl. Mix well to coat and refrigerate at least 1 hour or up to 8 hours.

2. Prepare the grill for medium-high heat.

3. Remove the chicken from the bowl and set on the grill rack coated with cooking spray. Grill 5 minutes per side, turning once. Brush the chicken with some of the peanut mixture, turn, and grill 1 minute. Brush chicken, turn, and grill 1 to 2 minutes longer or until a thermometer inserted into the thickest portion registers 165°F. Serve the chicken with the remaining sauce.

■ Eat One Serving:

397

CALORIES,
31 g protein, 21 g carbohydrates, 20 g fat, 3 g saturated fat, 63 mg cholesterol, 716 mg sodium*, 3 g fiber

A SINGLE SERVING OF THIS RECIPE COUNTS AS A FLAT BELLY DIET MEAL WITHOUT ANY ADD-ONS!

* Limit saturated fat to no more than 10% of total calories—about 20 grams for most men—and sodium intake to no more than 2,300 milligrams.

Grilled Chicken Thighs with Avocado Salsa

Preparation time: 15 minutes / Cooking time: 25 minutes / Makes 4 servings

1 teaspoon chili powder

½ teaspoon garlic powder

¼ teaspoon ground coriander

¾ teaspoon salt

¼ teaspoon black pepper

4 (4-ounce) bone-in skinless chicken thighs, trimmed

MUFA: 1 Hass avocado, peeled, pitted, and finely diced

3 plum tomatoes, seeded and chopped

1 small red onion, finely chopped

1 tablespoon lime juice

1 tablespoon chopped fresh cilantro

4 corn tortillas

1. Prepare the grill for indirect heat grilling.

2. Combine the chili powder, garlic powder, coriander, ½ teaspoon salt, and pepper in a bowl. Sprinkle the mixture over the chicken thighs to coat. Set the chicken on the grill rack coated with cooking spray, away from the heat source. Grill the chicken, turning occasionally, for 22 to 25 minutes, or until a thermometer inserted into the thickest portion registers 170°F.

3. Meanwhile, combine the avocado, tomato, onion, lime juice, cilantro, and remaining ¼ teaspoon salt in a bowl.

4. To serve, heat the tortillas on the grill over the heat source, turning occasionally, for 1 to 2 minutes, until slightly toasted. Serve the chicken with avocado salsa and tortillas.

■ Eat One Serving:

286

CALORIES,
18 g protein, 22 g carbohydrates, 14 g fat, 2.8 g saturated fat, 57 mg cholesterol, 530 mg sodium, 5 g fiber

MAKE IT A FLAT BELLY DIET MEAL:
Serve with ½ cup pinto beans (122).

■ Total Meal:

408

CALORIES

Pesto-Parmesan-Topped Burgers on Portuguese Rolls

Preparation time: 10 minutes / Cooking time: 10 minutes / Makes 4 servings

1 pound extra-lean ground beef

½ teaspoon salt

¼ teaspoon black pepper

2 tablespoons shredded Parmesan cheese

4 (1½-ounce) Portuguese rolls, split and toasted

4 Boston lettuce leaves

½ tomato, cut into 4 slices

MUFA: ¼ cup pesto

½ red onion, cut into 4 slices

1. Prepare the grill for medium-high heat.

2. Combine the beef, salt, and pepper in a bowl and mix gently. Form into four ½"-thick burger patties.

3. Set the burgers on the grill rack coated with cooking spray. Grill 4 minutes. Turn the burgers, grill 4 minutes longer, then top with Parmesan. Grill about 2 minutes longer, until cooked through and the Parmesan melts. Remove from the grill.

4. Set the roll bottoms on a work surface. Top each with 1 lettuce leaf, 1 tomato slice, 1 tablespoon pesto, 1 onion slice, and 1 burger. Top the burger with the other half of the roll.

■ **Eat One Serving:**

342

CALORIES,
29 g protein, 26 g carbohydrates, 14 g fat, 3.4 g saturated fat, 67 mg cholesterol, 794 mg sodium*, 2 g fiber

MAKE IT A FLAT BELLY DIET MEAL:
Serve with 1 cup baby carrots (53).

■ **Total Meal:**

395

CALORIES

* Limit saturated fat to no more than 10% of total calories—about 20 grams for most men—and sodium intake to no more than 2,300 milligrams.

Grilled Flank Steak with Olive Oil Mojo Sauce

Preparation time: 10 minutes / Cooking time: 12 minutes / Makes 4 servings

MUFA: ¼ cup olive oil

- ¼ cup orange juice
- ¼ cup chopped fresh cilantro
- ¼ cup chopped fresh basil
- 3 tablespoons lime juice
- 3 cloves garlic, minced
- 1 teaspoon freshly grated lime zest
- ¾ teaspoon ground cumin
- ¾ teaspoon salt
- 1 pound lean flank steak, trimmed
- ¼ teaspoon black pepper

1. Combine the oil, orange juice, cilantro, basil, lime juice, garlic, zest, cumin, and ½ teaspoon salt in a bowl. Combine the flank steak and 3 tablespoons oil mixture in a separate bowl, turning to coat. Refrigerate the steak at least 2 hours or up to 4 hours, turning occasionally.

2. Prepare the grill for medium-high heat.

3. Remove the steak from the bowl and sprinkle with the remaining ¼ teaspoon salt and pepper. Set on the grill rack coated with cooking spray. Grill, turning once, 10 to 12 minutes for medium-rare or until the desired level of doneness. Transfer to a cutting board and let stand 5 minutes. Thinly slice across the grain. Divide among 4 plates and spoon the remaining oil mixture over the steak.

■ **Eat One Serving:**

305

CALORIES,

25 g protein, 4 g carbohydrates, 21 g fat, 4.8 g saturated fat*, 48 mg cholesterol, 504 mg sodium, 0 g fiber

MAKE IT A FLAT BELLY DIET MEAL:

Serve with 1 cup of steamed broccoli florets (44) and 1 cup of steamed cauliflower florets (29).

■ **Total Meal:**

378

CALORIES

* Limit saturated fat to no more than 10% of total calories—about 20 grams for most men—and sodium intake to no more than 2,300 milligrams.

Grilled Filet Mignon with Grilled Onion and Avocado

Preparation time: 10 minutes / Cooking time: 25 minutes / Makes 4 servings

1 large red onion, cut into ½" slices

1 tablespoon olive oil

¾ teaspoon salt

¼ teaspoon black pepper

2 tomatoes, seeded and coarsely chopped

3 teaspoons lime juice

MUFA: 1 medium Hass avocado, peeled, pitted, and cut into 8 slices

4 (3-ounce) filet mignons

1. Prepare the grill for medium-high heat grilling.

2. Brush the onion slices with 1½ teaspoons oil and sprinkle with ¼ teaspoon salt and ⅛ teaspoon pepper. Set on the grill rack coated with cooking spray and grill 6 to 7 minutes per side, until well marked and tender. Transfer to a cutting board, coarsely chop, and toss in a bowl with the tomatoes, 2 teaspoons lime juice, and ⅛ teaspoon salt.

3. Sprinkle the avocado with ⅛ teaspoon salt and 1 teaspoon lime juice. Transfer to a plate and reserve. Brush the filet mignons with the remaining 1½ teaspoons oil and sprinkle with remaining ¼ teaspoon salt and ⅛ teaspoon pepper. Grill 3 to 4 minutes per side for medium-rare.

4. Set the filet mignons on each of 4 plates. Spoon the onion mixture onto the plates and top each with 2 avocado slices.

■ **Eat One Serving:**

258

CALORIES,
20 g protein, 8 g carbohydrates, 16 g fat, 3.7 g saturated fat, 61 mg cholesterol, 490 mg sodium, 8 g fiber

MAKE IT A FLAT BELLY DIET MEAL:
Serve with 1 large ear of corn (123).

■ **Total Meal:**

381

CALORIES

Marinated Grilled Boneless Pork Ribs

Preparation time: 10 minutes / Cooking time: 18-22 minutes / Makes 4 servings

MUFA: ¼ cup olive oil

¼ cup chopped fresh parsley

2 tablespoons fresh lemon juice

4 cloves garlic, minced

1 teaspoon crushed fennel seed

½ teaspoon ground cumin

1 pound lean country-style boneless loin pork ribs

½ teaspoon salt

¼ teaspoon black pepper

1. Combine the oil, parsley, lemon juice, garlic, fennel seed, and cumin in a large bowl. Transfer 2 tablespoons of the mixture to a small bowl and reserve. Add the ribs to the large bowl and toss well to coat. Refrigerate at least 4 hours or up to 8 hours, turning occasionally.

2. Prepare the grill for medium-high heat.

3. Remove the ribs from the bowl and sprinkle with salt and pepper. Set on the grill rack coated with cooking spray. Cook, turning once, 18 to 20 minutes, or until the thermometer reads 150° to 155°F. Brush the ribs with the remaining 2 tablespoons oil mixture and grill 2 minutes longer. Serve hot.

Eat One Serving:

CALORIES,
24 g protein, 2.3 g carbohydrates, 20 g fat, 4 g saturated fat*, 84 mg cholesterol, 371 mg sodium, 1 g fiber

MAKE IT A FLAT BELLY DIET MEAL:
Serve with 1 medium baked potato with skin (161).

Total Meal:

CALORIES

* Limit saturated fat to no more than 10% of total calories—about 20 grams for most men— and sodium intake to no more than 2,300 milligrams.

Mediterranean-Style Lamb Chops with Cucumber Salad

Preparation time: 10 minutes / Cooking time: 8 minutes / Makes 4 servings

4 (3-ounce) lean loin lamb chops, trimmed

MUFA: ¼ cup extra-virgin olive oil

3 cloves garlic, minced

1 teaspoon dried rosemary

3 plum tomatoes, seeded and sliced into strips

2 cucumbers, peeled, seeded, and sliced

½ fennel bulb, thinly sliced

⅓ red onion, thinly sliced

1 tablespoon red wine vinegar

½ teaspoon salt

¼ teaspoon black pepper

2 whole wheat pitas, halved crosswise

1. Combine the lamb, 1 tablespoon oil, garlic, and rosemary in a bowl. Refrigerate 30 minutes, turning occasionally.

2. Meanwhile, combine the tomatoes, cucumbers, fennel, onion, vinegar, ¼ teaspoon salt, ⅛ teaspoon pepper, and remaining 3 tablespoons oil in a bowl.

3. Prepare the grill for medium-high heat.

4. Remove the lamb from the bowl. Sprinkle with the remaining ¼ teaspoon salt and ⅛ teaspoon pepper. Set on the grill rack coated with cooking spray. Grill 3 to 4 minutes per side or until desired doneness. Serve with the cucumber salad. Toast the pitas and serve on the side.

Eat One Serving:

CALORIES,
22 g protein, 22 g carbohydrates, 20 g fat, 3.8 g saturated fat, 56 mg cholesterol, 524 mg sodium, 5 g fiber

MAKE IT A FLAT BELLY DIET MEAL:
Serve with 1 cup mandarin oranges (72).

Total Meal:

CALORIES

Lemon-Herb-Marinated Tuna Burger with Wasabi Aioli

Preparation time: 5 minutes / Cooking time: 4 minutes / Makes 4 servings

MUFA: ¼ cup canola oil mayonnaise

- 1 tablespoon lemon juice
- ½ clove garlic, minced
- ½ green onion, thinly sliced
- ¼ teaspoon prepared wasabi paste (not powdered)
- 4 (4-ounce) yellowfin tuna steaks
- 2 teaspoons Asian (toasted) sesame oil
- ¼ teaspoon salt
- 4 hamburger rolls
- 1 cup fresh arugula leaves
- ¼ medium cucumber, cut into 12 slices
- 8 slices pickled ginger (optional)

1. Prepare the grill for medium-high heat.

2. Combine the mayonnaise, lemon juice, garlic, onion, and wasabi paste in a bowl and mix well.

3. Brush the tuna steaks with the sesame oil and sprinkle with salt. Set on the grill rack coated with cooking spray. Grill 2 minutes per side or until well marked and cooked to the desired doneness.

4. Arrange the roll bottoms on each of 4 plates. Top each with ¼ cup arugula, 3 cucumber slices, 2 ginger slices, if using, and 1 tuna steak. Spread the top half of each roll with the mayonnaise mixture and set each on the tuna steak. Serve immediately.

■ **Eat One Serving:**

369

CALORIES,
32 g protein, 22 g carbohydrates, 17 g fat, 2.1 g saturated fat, 56 mg cholesterol, 505 mg sodium, 1 g fiber

A SINGLE SERVING OF THIS RECIPE COUNTS AS A FLAT BELLY DIET MEAL WITHOUT ANY ADD-ONS!

Asian-Marinated Grilled Tuna Steaks with Crunchy Peanut Dressing

Preparation time: 5 minutes / Cooking time: 6 minutes / Makes 4 servings

²/₃ cup orange juice

¼ cup lemon juice

3 tablespoons low-sodium soy sauce

3 tablespoons grated fresh ginger

2 cloves garlic, minced

4 (6-ounce) tuna steaks

MUFA: ½ cup unsalted peanuts, chopped

¼ cup seasoned rice vinegar

1½ tablespoons honey

1 tablespoon mirin

6 cups mixed greens

1. Combine the orange juice, lemon juice, soy sauce, ginger, and garlic in a large bowl and mix well. Add the tuna steaks and refrigerate 30 minutes, turning occasionally.

2. Meanwhile, combine the peanuts, vinegar, honey, and mirin in a bowl and mix well.

3. Prepare the grill for medium-high heat.

4. Remove the tuna steaks from the marinade and set on the grill rack coated with cooking spray. Grill 3 minutes per side, brushing with the remaining marinade, or until well marked and cooked to the desired doneness.

5. Arrange 1½ cups greens on each of 4 plates. Top each with a tuna steak. Spoon the peanut mixture over the steaks and greens.

Eat One Serving:

375 CALORIES, 47 g protein, 22 g carbohydrates, 11 g fat, 1.7 g saturated fat, 76 g cholesterol, 541 mg sodium, 4 g fiber

A SINGLE SERVING OF THIS RECIPE COUNTS AS A FLAT BELLY DIET MEAL WITHOUT ANY ADD-ONS!

Grilled Salmon with Herbs, Dijon, and Extra-Virgin Olive Oil

Preparation time: 10 minutes / Cooking time: 12 minutes / Makes 4 servings

MUFA: ¼ cup extra-virgin olive oil

- ¼ cup chopped fresh basil
- ¼ cup chopped fresh parsley
- 2 tablespoons lemon juice
- 1 tablespoon Dijon mustard
- 1 clove garlic, minced
- ¼ teaspoon salt
- 4 (4-ounce) skinless salmon fillets
- ¼ teaspoon black pepper

1. Combine the oil, basil, parsley, lemon juice, mustard, garlic, and salt in a bowl. Combine the salmon and 2 tablespoons oil mixture in a separate bowl. Refrigerate 30 minutes, turning occasionally.

2. Prepare the grill for medium-high heat.

3. Sprinkle the salmon with pepper and set on the grill rack coated generously with cooking spray. Grill 5 to 6 minutes per side, or until the fish flakes easily with a fork.

4. Set the salmon on serving plates and spoon the remaining oil mixture over each piece before serving.

■ **Eat One Serving:**

343

CALORIES, 23 g protein, 2 g carbohydrates, 26 g fat, 4.4 g saturated fat*, 67 mg cholesterol, 305 mg sodium, 0 g fiber

MAKE IT A FLAT BELLY DIET MEAL: Serve with ½ pound (approximately 2 cups) of grilled asparagus spears (46).

■ **Total Meal:**

389

CALORIES

* Limit saturated fat to no more than 10% of total calories—about 20 grams for most men— and sodium intake to no more than 2,300 milligrams.

Balsamic Portobello and Vegetable Mixed Grill

Preparation time: 15 minutes / Cooking time: 20 minutes / Makes 4 servings

MUFA: ¼ cup extra-virgin olive oil

2 tablespoons balsamic vinegar

1 teaspoon dried basil

1 teaspoon dried oregano

4 medium portobello mushroom caps

1 pound asparagus, trimmed

1 (10- to 12-ounce) zucchini, cut diagonally into 12 slices

1 large Vidalia or other sweet onion, cut into 4 slices

¾ teaspoon salt

¼ teaspoon black pepper

4 ounces Italian bread, sliced

1. Prepare the grill for medium-high heat.

2. Combine the oil, vinegar, basil, and oregano in a bowl. Brush the mushrooms, asparagus, zucchini, and onion with the oil mixture. Sprinkle with salt and pepper.

3. Set the mushrooms, asparagus, zucchini, and onion slices on the grill rack coated with cooking spray. Grill the vegetables until crisp-tender and well marked, 7 to 8 minutes for the asparagus, 5 to 6 minutes per side for the zucchini, 7 to 8 minutes per side for the onion, and 8 to 9 minutes per side for the mushrooms. Serve with sliced Italian bread.

■ **Eat One Serving:**

302

CALORIES,

9 g protein, 34 g carbohydrates, 16 g fat, 2.2 g saturated fat, 0 mg cholesterol, 627 mg sodium*, 6 g fiber

MAKE IT A FLAT BELLY DIET MEAL:

Serve with 1 cup fresh blueberries (82).

■ **Total Meal:**

384

CALORIES

* Limit saturated fat to no more than 10% of total calories—about 20 grams for most men—and sodium intake to no more than 2,300 milligrams.

Chili-Spiced Fries with Chipotle Ketchup

Preparation time: 10 minutes / Cooking time: 27 minutes / Makes 4 servings

2 teaspoons chili powder
½ teaspoon ground cumin
¼ teaspoon salt
½ cup ketchup
½ teaspoon ground chipotle pepper
3 russet potatoes, 1¼ pounds, cut into 16 wedges each

MUFA: ¼ cup olive oil

1. Preheat the oven to 450°F. Coat 2 large-rimmed baking sheets with cooking spray.

2. Combine the chili powder, cumin, and salt in a large bowl. Combine the ketchup and ground chipotle in a separate bowl.

3. Combine the potatoes and 3 tablespoons of the oil in a large bowl, tossing well to coat. Arrange the potatoes in a single layer on the baking sheets. Pour any oil left in the bowl over the potatoes.

4. Bake 15 minutes, turn the potatoes and bake 12 minutes longer or until golden brown and crisp. Add to the bowl with the chili powder and toss well. Drizzle the fries with the remaining tablespoon of oil. Serve with the ketchup mixture.

■ **Eat One Serving:**

262

CALORIES,
3 g protein, 34 g carbohydrates, 14 g fat, 1.9 g saturated fat, 0 mg cholesterol, 533 mg sodium, 2 g fiber

MAKE IT A FLAT BELLY DIET MEAL:
Serve with 3 ounces roasted chicken breast (140).

■ **Total Meal:**

402

CALORIES

Mexican Bean and Avocado Salsa with Baked Tortilla Chips

Preparation time: 15 minutes / Makes 4 servings

1 (15-ounce) can no-salt-added black beans, drained and rinsed

MUFA: 1 Hass avocado, peeled, pitted, and diced

1 small white onion, finely chopped

2 plum tomatoes, seeded and chopped

1 jalapeño pepper, finely chopped

2 tablespoons chopped fresh cilantro

1 tablespoon lime juice

½ teaspoon salt

4 ounces baked tortilla chips

Combine the beans, avocado, onion, tomato, jalapeño, cilantro, lime juice, and salt in a bowl and mix well. Serve with tortilla chips.

■ **Eat One Serving:**

240

CALORIES,
8 g protein, 39 g carbohydrates, 7 g fat, 1 g saturated fat, 0 mg cholesterol, 647 mg sodium*, 8 g fiber

MAKE IT A FLAT BELLY DIET MEAL:
Serve with 1 cup of papaya (54) and 1 cup of mango (108), mixed.

■ **Total Meal:**

402

CALORIES

* Limit saturated fat to no more than 10% of total calories—about 20 grams for most men—and sodium intake to no more than 2,300 milligrams.

POWER SNACKS & SIDES

Sautéed Spinach with Garlic and Red-Pepper Flakes

Preparation time: 5 minutes / Cooking time: 5 minutes Makes 4 servings

MUFA: ¼ cup extra-virgin olive oil

- 4 cloves garlic, thinly sliced
- ⅛ teaspoon crushed red-pepper flakes
- 2 (9-ounce) bags prewashed spinach
- ¼ teaspoon salt

1. Heat the oil in a large nonstick skillet over medium-high heat. Add the garlic and red-pepper flakes and cook, stirring occasionally, about 1 minute, until the garlic is lightly browned.
2. Add 1 bag of spinach and cook, turning with kitchen tongs, until wilted. Add the remaining bag of spinach and cook, turning, 1 to 2 minutes, until wilted and hot. Sprinkle with salt and divide among 4 plates.

■ **Eat One Serving:**

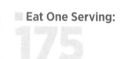

CALORIES,
6 g protein, 8 g carbohydrates, 15 g fat, 2 g saturated fat, 0 mg cholesterol, 297 mg sodium, 4 g fiber

MAKE IT A FLAT BELLY DIET MEAL:
Serve with 3 ounces roasted center-cut pork loin (199).
■ **Total Meal:**

374

CALORIES

Macadamia Nut Blondies

Preparation time: 10 minutes / Cooling time: 30 minutes / Makes 8 servings

1 cup all-purpose flour

1½ teaspoons baking powder

¼ teaspoon salt

6 tablespoons trans-free margarine, melted

2 eggs, lightly beaten

1 cup packed light brown sugar

1½ teaspoons pure vanilla extract

MUFA: 1 cup unsalted dry-roasted macadamia nuts, coarsely chopped

1. Preheat the oven to 350°F. Coat an 8" x 8" baking pan with cooking spray and dust lightly with flour.

2. Combine the flour, baking powder, and salt in a bowl. Combine the margarine, eggs, sugar, and vanilla in a separate bowl. Stir the flour mixture into the margarine mixture until well combined. Stir in the macadamia nuts. Pour into the prepared baking pan.

3. Bake 24 to 25 minutes, or until a toothpick inserted into the center comes out with a few moist crumbs. Remove from the oven and cool in the pan on a wire rack for 30 minutes. Cut into 8 or 16 squares and serve.

■ **Eat One Serving:**

364

CALORIES,
5 g protein, 42 g carbohydrates, 20 g fat, 3.1 g saturated fat, 55 mg cholesterol, 245 mg sodium, 2 g fiber

MAKE IT A FLAT BELLY DIET MEAL:
Serve with ½ cup of fat-free milk (42).

■ **Total Meal:**

406

CALORIES

Dark Chocolate Pudding

Preparation time: 5 minutes / Cooking time: 10 minutes / Makes 4 servings

2 cups fat-free milk

½ cup packed dark brown sugar

2 tablespoons unsweetened cocoa powder

2 tablespoons cornstarch

MUFA: 4 ounces semisweet chocolate, chopped

1½ teaspoons pure vanilla extract

1. Whisk together the milk, sugar, cocoa powder, and cornstarch in a medium saucepan. Bring to a boil, stirring, over medium heat and boil for 1 minute. Remove from the heat and add the chocolate and vanilla, stirring until smooth.

2. Divide among 4 small custard cups or bowls. Press a piece of plastic wrap directly onto the pudding and cool to room temperature. Chill at least 2 hours before serving.

■ **Eat One Serving:**

312

CALORIES,

7 g protein, 56 g carbohydrates, 9 g fat, 5.2 g saturated fat*, 2 mg cholesterol, 60 mg sodium, 2 g fiber

MAKE IT A FLAT BELLY DIET MEAL:
Serve with 1 medium banana (105).

■ **Total Meal:**

417

CALORIES

* Limit saturated fat to no more than 10% of total calories—about 20 grams for most men— and sodium intake to no more than 2,300 milligrams.

Cashew Chocolate Chip Cookie Ice Cream Sandwiches

Preparation time: 15 minutes / Makes 4 servings

2 cups slow-churned low-fat vanilla ice cream, softened

MUFA: ½ cup lightly salted dry-roasted cashews

16 reduced-fat chocolate chip cookies

Combine the ice cream and cashews in a bowl. Fold together with a wooden spoon or rubber spatula. Arrange 8 cookies, bottom side up, on a work surface. Spoon the ice cream mixture onto the cookies. Top with the remaining cookies, bottom side down, pressing slightly to form a sandwich. Smooth the sides with a spoon and set on a plate or small baking sheet. Freeze for 2 hours before serving.

■ **Eat One Serving:**

385

CALORIES,
7 g protein, 51 g carbohydrates, 18 g fat, 5.5 g saturated fat*, 20 mg cholesterol, 234 mg sodium, 2 g fiber

A SINGLE SERVING OF THIS RECIPE COUNTS AS A FLAT BELLY DIET MEAL WITHOUT ANY ADD-ONS!

* Limit saturated fat to no more than 10% of total calories—about 20 grams for most men—and sodium intake to no more than 2,300 milligrams.

DESSERTS

Strawberry-Banana and Pecan Sundaes

Preparation time: 10 minutes / Cooking time: 5 minutes / Makes 4 servings

MUFA: ½ cup pecan halves, chopped

- 1 tablespoon trans-free margarine
- 2 bananas, sliced
- 3 cups fresh strawberries, sliced
- 3 tablespoons sugar
- 2 cups slow-churned low-fat vanilla ice cream
- 4 maraschino cherries

1. Heat the pecans, shaking often, in a medium nonstick skillet over medium-high heat until lightly toasted. Transfer to a bowl and cool for 5 minutes.

2. Return the skillet to the stove and melt the margarine over medium heat. Add the bananas, strawberries, and sugar and cook, stirring occasionally, for about 2 minutes, or until just softened and warm.

3. Scoop ½ cup ice cream into each of 4 sundae glasses and top with one-quarter of the fruit and 2 tablespoons pecans. Top each with 1 maraschino cherry. Serve immediately.

■ **Eat One Serving:**

363

CALORIES,

6 g protein, 53 g carbohydrates, 16 g fat, 3.4 g saturated fat, 37 mg cholesterol, 73 mg sodium, 5 g fiber

MAKE IT A FLAT BELLY DIET MEAL:

Drizzle with 1 tablespoon chocolate syrup (55).

■ **Total Meal:**

418

CALORIES

Cinnamon Apple Crisp

Preparation time: 15 minutes / Cooking time: 40 minutes / Makes 6 servings

2 pounds golden delicious apples, peeled, cored, thinly sliced

$^2/_3$ cup packed light brown sugar

$^1/_2$ cup all-purpose flour

1 teaspoon ground cinnamon

1 teaspoon pure vanilla extract

1 cup oatmeal

$^1/_8$ teaspoon salt

3 tablespoons trans-free margarine, cut into small pieces

MUFA: $^3/_4$ **cup walnuts, coarsely chopped**

1. Preheat the oven to 375°F. Coat an 8" x 8" baking dish with cooking spray.

2. Combine the apples, $^1/_3$ cup sugar, 2 tablespoons flour, $^1/_2$ teaspoon cinnamon, and vanilla in a bowl and toss well. Pour into the prepared baking dish. Combine the oatmeal, salt, and the remaining $^1/_3$ cup sugar, 6 tablespoons flour, $^1/_2$ teaspoon cinnamon in a separate bowl. Add the margarine and crumble until well incorporated. Stir in the walnuts and sprinkle over the apples.

3. Bake, uncovered, 35 to 40 minutes, or until the fruit is tender and bubbly and the topping is lightly browned. Let cool on a rack for 30 minutes before serving.

■ **Eat One Serving:**

354

CALORIES,
5 g protein, 58 g carbohydrates, 13 g fat, 1.4 g saturated fat, 2 mg cholesterol, 101 mg sodium, 5 g fiber

MAKE IT A FLAT BELLY DIET MEAL:
Serve with $^1/_4$ cup of Breyers Natural Vanilla ice cream (65).

■ **Total Meal:**

419

CALORIES

READ A FLAT BELLY
SUCCESS
STORY

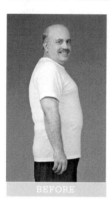

BEFORE

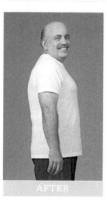

AFTER

Phil
DiScala

AGE: 54

POUNDS LOST:

9.2

IN 32 DAYS

ALL-OVER
INCHES LOST:

8.6

2.25 FROM
THE WAIST

↘ **favorite
mini meal**
Savory Turkey
Pasta, *page 127*

**"Do you have any idea
how good it feels to put
on a suit I haven't worn
in over 4 years?"** Phil
DiScala beamed as he asked this
question during his final Flat Belly
weigh in. And he had good reason to
feel proud! Losing 9.2 pounds and 8.6
inches, Phil not only changed his suit
size—he changed his life. According to
the Flat Belly bioelectrical impedance
measurements, he also gained 10
pounds of muscle. That's a plus in the
weight loss arena since muscle burns
more calories than fat . . . even when
you're sleeping!

Phil, a 54-year-old senior specialist
for a utilities company in New York
City, has a fairly sedentary job, and
over the years he ate too much,
exercised too little, and ballooned to
an unhealthy (and uncomfortable) 250
pounds. Phil had tried other weight
loss plans and would drop a few
pounds, but then grew tired of
counting calories and feeling hungry.
Eventually, he'd drop the plan and
gain back the weight.

Now, thanks to the Flat Belly Diet
for Men, Phil has changed his ways
permanently. Phil says, "With the Flat
Belly Diet, I feel full and have a lot
more energy. I don't look at it as a
'diet,' but rather a better lifestyle of
eating and exercise." So instead of
ordering fried foods, he's opting for
baked, steamed, or grilled items. And
instead of engulfing huge plates of

pasta, he's enjoying more reasonable portions mixed with filling and tasty MUFAs. "I love pasta," says Phil. "And now I enjoy it in smaller quantities with a MUFA, like extra-virgin olive oil. The fat is flavorful and satisfying, so I need a lot less of the pasta." Phil also takes advantage of the Flat Belly Diet for Men "free foods" by having generous salads with dark leafy greens, tomatoes, and cucumbers. Having large portions of lower-calorie items helps him feel fuller, longer.

Phil has not only improved his eating habits, he has also increased his activity—significantly. "This is my schedule: stationary bike 5 to 7 miles a day and mix the Pilates workout with a general strength-training workout. I do that three times a week." In fact, as an experienced (though out of practice) street biker, he is thrilled to have the energy and mobility to get back on a bike and to improve his 5-mile bike time by 15 minutes!

And Phil is enjoying these lifestyle changes together with his supportive wife, Theresa. They eat their meals at the same time and exercise as a team whenever possible.

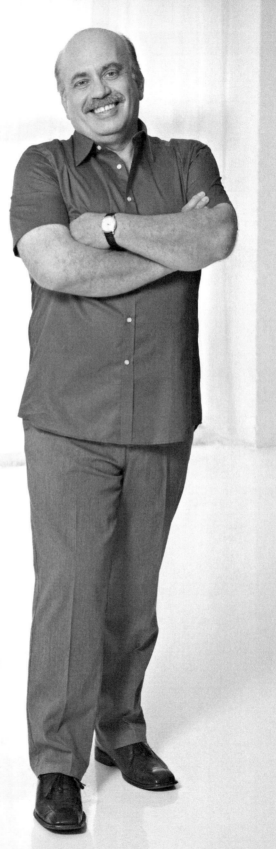

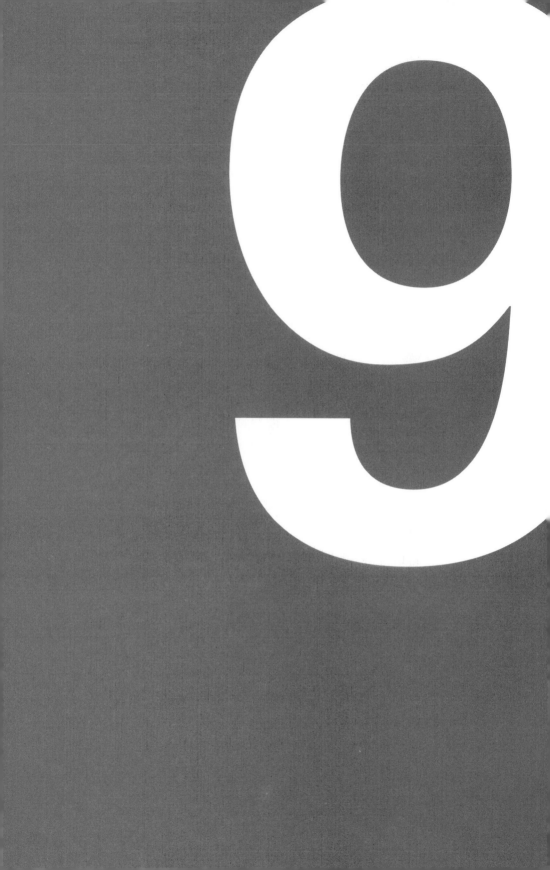

THE FLAT BELLY DIET
FOR MEN
WORKOUT

YOU'VE SPENT FAR too long holding in your gut trying to impress people. It's about time that your gut—and the rest of your body—did something about making you look more impressive.

That's where the right exercise plan can help. Even though you'll see remarkable weight loss results by simply following the diet plan, performing the right workout program, along with eating the Flat Belly way, can make it even easier to shed those unwanted pounds and get six-pack abs.

If it's been a while since your waistline was trim and cut, not to worry because you're not alone. We've all been there. It's not easy juggling work, family, and a myriad of other responsibilities 24/7. And with so many people depending on you, the thought of finding the time to change your diet—let alone take on an exercise program—might seem a bit overwhelming. But it's worth it! Especially if you want to see better results in far less time.

The Science That Gets Results!

I asked fitness expert Myatt Murphy, author of *The Body You Want in the Time You Have*, *The Men's Health Gym Bible*, and *Men's Health Ultimate Dumbbell Guide*, to devise a companion workout to the Flat Belly Diet for Men—one that would work best to meet a man's needs.

▇ **To make it doable,** he kept the exercise plan simple, sticking with cardio that only takes a pair of walking shoes, plus a strength-training program that requires nothing more than a pair of dumbbells and a floor mat. No benches, machines, or fancy gym memberships necessary.

▇ **To make it functional,** he incorporated moves that leave your muscles no choice but to work together. As you burn fat and build muscle, you'll also be making more of a mind-body connection, and that means more power, speed, and balance when moving in any direction—whether that's on the field, on the job, or working away at home.

▇ **To make it practical,** he chose a series of techniques that have been scientifically shown to help burn more fat in a shorter period of time.

There's a reason why you can't seem to bring your belly down to the size you wish it would be. But with all three of these principles in place, that's all about to change, courtesy of the following three-part workout routine.

The Flat Belly Workout Basics

THE ROUTINE YOU'LL BE following is a 28-day plan that incorporates three specific components:

1. CARDIOVASCULAR EXERCISE to melt fat, burn through excess calories, and lower your blood pressure

2. **WEIGHT TRAINING** to build and preserve muscle so you will burn more calories all day long

3. **CORE STRENGTH-FOCUSED ABDOMINAL EXERCISES** that firm and flatten your midsection

To burn off as much belly fat as possible, the first portion of the program will incorporate cardiovascular exercise into your weekly routine. If you have access to cardiovascular equipment—such as a treadmill, stair climber, or bicycle—or prefer to work up a sweat playing sports, that's entirely fine. However, an equally effective (and inexpensive) way to shed those excess pounds is walking.

If you're like most guys, you're probably thinking that walking is just too easy to be considered a *real* workout, but that's a huge misconception. Not only have countless studies shown that regular walking can lower blood pressure and strengthen the heart and lungs, but it's also a very effective tool to burn calories and body fat.

The truth is, your body doesn't keep score whether you're walking, running, shooting hoops, or throwing the football. It responds to effort and exertion. The type of exercise or activity you do to make those two things happen is irrelevant. Any activity that raises your heart rate and maintains it for at least 20 minutes can improve your cardiovascular abilities significantly and burn fat. And what makes walking so beneficial is that you can do it for a long time. Research shows that your body begins to burn a larger percentage of stored fat (instead of stored glycogen) after 20 minutes of cardiovascular exercise. Most high-impact activities can tire you out before you hit this zone, but walking lets you exercise long past the 20-minute mark so you tap into more of your stored fat.

The trick is to make it challenging enough to get the results you want. That's why we've designed two specific types of walking programs to double your results: the **Fat Blast Walk** and the **Calorie Torch Walk**.

Three days a week, you'll do the Fat Blast Walk, where you'll walk at a moderately brisk pace for a longer duration, which has been shown to trigger your body to burn more stored body fat. You'll walk for a longer time as your body acclimates to getting fitter.

In between those days, you'll perform the Calorie Torch Walk, a unique interval-training routine where you'll alternate between walking briskly with walking at a faster, higher-intensity pace. Research shows that this type of training not only keeps your metabolism revved for a longer time after you exercise (so you burn even more calories at rest), but it also prevents your body from breaking down any of your hard-earned muscle as fuel, perfect for the guy who is concerned about losing muscle while losing weight.

To build muscle, firm your belly, and rev up your metabolism, you'll also be adding a weight-training routine (the **Maximum Metabolism Workout**) and an abdominal exercise routine (the **Cut to the Core Routine**).

The Maximum Metabolism Workout combines four multijoint exercises that train several muscles to work together instead of isolating just one, giving you the best full-body workout in the shortest time possible. The more muscles you can work at once, the more calories your body has to burn. Plus, all of these moves require a certain amount of balance, which forces your abs to constantly engage as you exercise, so they're always working behind the scenes.

Finally, the Cut to the Core Routine mixes five of the most effective abdominal exercises into one plan that hits every part of your midsection. These moves have been shown to be more efficient at activating your abdominal muscles than the traditional crunch by as much as 140 percent, making it easier to firm your waistline in far less time.

So where's the added "guy edge" to these two strength-training routines? That's easy. One, most men tend to fall into the habit of being muscularly imbalanced, due in part to focusing too much on the muscles they can see and too little on the muscles they can't. It's the reason many older men tend not to be as well proportioned as they should be and suffer from a higher risk of injury. This workout helps correct those flaws by training both sides—front and back—equally, ensuring you'll hit more muscle groups in every workout for a more balanced physique (above and below your waistline).

Two, it's designed to improve your performance—on and off the field or just in everyday life. Explosive movements incorporated into this program, such as jumping, sprinting, or throwing, require all of your muscles to be in sync with each other. Whether you need your muscles to work more efficiently together so you can catch a fastball or simply catch a taxi, these exercises use a combination of compound moves that help develop functional strength and improve performance and body awareness.

Just like the two walking programs, you'll aim for doing each of these routines three times a week, alternating between them every other day. The reason you need to switch is to give your muscles a chance to rest. However, if you find working out six times a week is too much to fit into your schedule, you can always miss a few. The same goes for the walking routines. But remember, the closer you stick to the complete three-part plan, the faster you'll shrink that belly and see the muscles you have hiding beneath.

The Intensity Is Up to You

To GET THE MOST from your walking workouts, you have to know how to push yourself. This means getting your heart pumping at a pace that's ideal for burning fat as efficiently as possible. Both the Fat Blast and the Calorie Torch walks accomplish that, but in two different ways.

For the Fat Blast Walk, you'll warm up walking at a low intensity, then begin walking at a moderately intense, brisk pace for a certain amount of time. Each week, you'll increase, the length of time you walk throughout the 28-day program. For the Calorie Torch Walk, you'll also warm up walking at a low intensity, then you'll walk at two different speeds, switching back and forth from a moderately intense, brisk pace to a faster, high-intensity pace.

So what exactly is a "brisk" or "fast" pace? What is the right speed that's considered low, moderate, or high intensity? Well, we can't give you an exact speed to stick with because that can differ from guy to guy. What may be moderately intense for one guy may be too easy (or too difficult) for another. Some researchers have tried to put a number to it. In fact, in a recent study published in the *American Journal of Preventive Medicine*, researchers at San Diego State University found that walking at a pace of 100 steps per minute (on level terrain) helps the average man reach a level of moderate intensity (which is roughly the intensity you will experience from walking at a brisk pace).[1] You can try that if you like, but there's another effective way to figure out if you're exercising hard enough. Here's how the levels of intensity break down:

	HOW IT FEELS	INTENSITY LEVEL	SPEED (MPH) *
WARMUP, COOLDOWN	Easy enough that you can belt out "The Star-Spangled Banner"	3–4 (LOW INTENSITY)	3.0–3.5
BRISK	You can talk, but singing's out of the question	5–6 (MODERATE INTENSITY)	3.5–4.0
FAST	You can blurt out brief phrases, but would rather not	7–8 (HIGH INTENSITY)	4.0+

*Note that these walking speeds are merely guidelines. Depending on your weight, fitness level, the evenness of the ground you're walking on, etc., these speeds may vary. Still, you can use these speeds to gauge if you're walking at the right intensity level that's recommended in both the Fat Blast and Calorie Torch workouts.

■ **FAT BLAST**—Steady-paced walks burn off belly fat. Walk at a brisk speed (5–6 intensity level).

■ **CALORIE TORCH**—Interval walks raise your calorie burn during and after your workout to shed even more belly fat. Alternate brisk walking (5–6 intensity level) with short bursts of fast walking (7–8 intensity level).

Some weeks you'll notice that more time will be added to your walks. There's a good reason for that. Your heart, muscles, and lungs will become stronger with each passing week. The problem? The stronger they become, the less taxing your workouts will be, which means you'll burn fewer calories overall. To keep your entire body constantly challenged, you'll add extra minutes to each workout for Weeks 2 and 3. That way, the intensity will stay at a high enough level to maximize your fat-burning potential. Once you reach Week 3, the two walking workouts are pretty intense, which is why you'll use the same recommended routine for Week 4 as well.

One-Minute Massage!

Whether you're new to exercise or not, the intensity of both walking workouts may make your hamstrings—the muscles along the backs of your thighs—feel tight and sore the next day. To get them loose and always ready to go, this massage-stretch can iron out the kinks so you stay on track every day.

■ Right after your walk, sit with your back and butt flat against a wall. Bend your left leg so that your left foot is flat on the floor. (Your right leg should stay extended straight in front of you.)

■ Make a fist with your left hand and place it behind your left knee, palm facing your hamstrings. Press in with your palm and run your fist down your thigh toward your butt 3 to 4 times.

■ Gently pull your left knee in toward your chest—holding your ankle with your right hand and your knee with your left hand—and pause for 2 to 3 seconds. Repeat this three-part cycle 2 to 3 times, then switch positions to loosen up your right leg.

The 1-Month Cardio Plan

	WEEK ONE		

DAY 1

FAT BLAST WALK

TOTAL WORKOUT TIME	THE BREAKDOWN	INTENSITY
30 minutes	3 minutes warmup	3–4
	25 minutes brisk	5–6
	2 minutes cooldown	3–4

DAY 2

CALORIE TORCH WALK

TOTAL WORKOUT TIME	THE BREAKDOWN	INTENSITY
25 minutes	3 minutes warmup	3–4
	4 minutes brisk	5–6
	1 minute fast (do brisk/fast intervals 4 times)	7–8
	2 minutes cooldown	3–4

DAY 3

FAT BLAST WALK

TOTAL WORKOUT TIME	THE BREAKDOWN	INTENSITY
30 minutes	3 minutes warmup	3–4
	25 minutes brisk	5–6
	2 minutes cooldown	3–4

DAY 4

CALORIE TORCH WALK

TOTAL WORKOUT TIME	THE BREAKDOWN	INTENSITY
25 minutes	3 minutes warmup	3–4
	4 minutes brisk	5–6
	1 minute fast (do brisk/fast intervals 4 times)	7–8
	2 minutes cooldown	3–4

DAY 5

FAT BLAST WALK

TOTAL WORKOUT TIME	THE BREAKDOWN	INTENSITY
30 minutes	3 minutes warmup	3–4
	25 minutes brisk	5–6
	2 minutes cooldown	3–4

DAY 6

CALORIE TORCH WALK

TOTAL WORKOUT TIME	THE BREAKDOWN	INTENSITY
25 minutes	3 minutes warmup	3–4
	4 minutes brisk	5–6
	1 minute fast (do brisk/fast intervals 4 times)	7–8
	2 minutes cooldown	3–4

DAY 7

REST

	WEEK TWO		

FAT BLAST WALK

DAY 1

TOTAL WORKOUT TIME	THE BREAKDOWN	INTENSITY
45 minutes	3 minutes warmup	3–4
	40 minutes brisk	5–6
	2 minutes cooldown	3–4

CALORIE TORCH WALK

DAY 2

TOTAL WORKOUT TIME	THE BREAKDOWN	INTENSITY
35 minutes	3 minutes warmup	3–4
	4 minutes brisk	5–6
	1 minute fast (do brisk/fast intervals 6 times)	7–8
	2 minutes cooldown	3–4

FAT BLAST WALK

DAY 3

TOTAL WORKOUT TIME	THE BREAKDOWN	INTENSITY
45 minutes	3 minutes warmup	3–4
	40 minutes brisk	5–6
	2 minutes cooldown	3–4

CALORIE TORCH WALK

DAY 4

TOTAL WORKOUT TIME	THE BREAKDOWN	INTENSITY
35 minutes	3 minutes warmup	3–4
	4 minutes brisk	5–6
	1 minute fast (do brisk/fast intervals 6 times)	7–8
	2 minutes cooldown	3–4

FAT BLAST WALK

DAY 5

TOTAL WORKOUT TIME	THE BREAKDOWN	INTENSITY
45 minutes	3 minutes warmup	3–4
	40 minutes brisk	5–6
	2 minutes cooldown	3–4

CALORIE TORCH WALK

DAY 6

TOTAL WORKOUT TIME	THE BREAKDOWN	INTENSITY
35 minutes	3 minutes warmup	3–4
	4 minutes brisk	5–6
	1 minute fast (do brisk/fast intervals 6 times)	7–8
	2 minutes cooldown	3–4

DAY 7

REST

FAT BLAST WALK

DAY 1

TOTAL WORKOUT TIME	THE BREAKDOWN	INTENSITY
60 minutes	3 minutes warmup	3–4
	55 minutes brisk	5–6
	2 minutes cooldown	3–4

CALORIE TORCH WALK

DAY 2

TOTAL WORKOUT TIME	THE BREAKDOWN	INTENSITY
45 minutes	3 minutes warmup	3–4
	4 minutes brisk	5–6
	1 minute fast (do brisk/fast intervals 8 times)	7–8
	2 minutes cooldown	3–4

FAT BLAST WALK

DAY 3

TOTAL WORKOUT TIME	THE BREAKDOWN	INTENSITY
60 minutes	3 minutes warmup	3–4
	55 minutes brisk	5–6
	2 minutes cooldown	3–4

CALORIE TORCH WALK

DAY 4

TOTAL WORKOUT TIME	THE BREAKDOWN	INTENSITY
45 minutes	3 minutes warmup	3–4
	4 minutes brisk	5–6
	1 minute fast (do brisk/fast intervals 8 times)	7–8
	2 minutes cooldown	3–4

FAT BLAST WALK

DAY 5

TOTAL WORKOUT TIME	THE BREAKDOWN	INTENSITY
60 minutes	3 minutes warmup	3–4
	55 minutes brisk	5–6
	2 minutes cooldown	3–4

CALORIE TORCH WALK

DAY 6

TOTAL WORKOUT TIME	THE BREAKDOWN	INTENSITY
45 minutes	3 minutes warmup	3–4
	4 minutes brisk	5–6
	1 minute fast (do brisk/fast intervals 8 times)	7–8
	2 minutes cooldown	3–4

DAY 7

REST

DAY 1

FAT BLAST WALK

TOTAL WORKOUT TIME	THE BREAKDOWN	INTENSITY
60 minutes	3 minutes warmup	3–4
	55 minutes brisk	5–6
	2 minutes cooldown	3–4

DAY 2

CALORIE TORCH WALK

TOTAL WORKOUT TIME	THE BREAKDOWN	INTENSITY
45 minutes	3 minutes warmup	3–4
	4 minutes brisk	5–6
	1 minute fast (do brisk/fast intervals 8 times)	7–8
	2 minutes cooldown	3–4

DAY 3

FAT BLAST WALK

TOTAL WORKOUT TIME	THE BREAKDOWN	INTENSITY
60 minutes	3 minutes warmup	3–4
	55 minutes brisk	5–6
	2 minutes cooldown	3–4

DAY 4

CALORIE TORCH WALK

TOTAL WORKOUT TIME	THE BREAKDOWN	INTENSITY
45 minutes	3 minutes warmup	3–4
	4 minutes brisk	5–6
	1 minute fast (do brisk/fast intervals 8 times)	7–8
	2 minutes cooldown	3–4

DAY 5

FAT BLAST WALK

TOTAL WORKOUT TIME	THE BREAKDOWN	INTENSITY
60 minutes	3 minutes warmup	3–4
	55 minutes brisk	5–6
	2 minutes cooldown	3–4

DAY 6

CALORIE TORCH WALK

TOTAL WORKOUT TIME	THE BREAKDOWN	INTENSITY
45 minutes	3 minutes warmup	3–4
	4 minutes brisk	5–6
	1 minute fast (do brisk/fast intervals 8 times)	7–8
	2 minutes cooldown	3–4

DAY 7

REST

Walk the Right Way

WALKING MAY BURN CALORIES, but to maximize your results and achieve the most fat-burning benefits, the trick is to learn how to do it as efficiently as possible.

First, walk tall by keeping yourself as upright as possible. Imagine trying to form a straight line from your ears through your shoulders and down to your hips. This will prevent you from leaning too far forward (an angle that can inhibit your lungs from expanding and delivering more oxygen throughout the body) or too far backward (an angle that can compromise the muscles of your lower back). Best rule of thumb: Just keep your eyes focused in front of you and your chin lifted as you walk. This should help naturally pull the shoulders back to prevent any slouching.

Next, keep the length of your stride as natural as possible. Trying to take longer steps won't help you burn additional calories. Instead, it will only change your natural rhythm, which can put stress on your hips. Finally, bend your arms

Gear Up for Your Walks

YOUR SHOES

Find a knowledgeable salesperson. Unlike mass-market retailers, specialty stores often employ trained shoe fitters who will ask you about your walking habits and watch you walk. This information will improve your chances of getting the right shoe for your feet.

Get your feet measured. Your size can change over time, and footwear that's too small can set you up for an array of problems. Make sure you have a thumb's width of room in front of the end of your big toe while you're standing rather than sitting.

Replace your shoes every 300 to 500 miles. That's about every 5 to 8 months if you're walking about 3 miles 5 days a week. By the time a sneaker looks trashed on the outside, the inside support and cushioning are long gone.

YOUR SOCKS

Look for synthetic fabrics that wick moisture away, keeping your feet dry and making them less prone to blisters. Avoid all-cotton socks. Since some are thick and others are thin, wear your walking socks when you try shoes on, because they can affect the fit.

at 90-degree angles and swing them about 7 to 8 inches forward from the body (no higher than chest level). As you draw them back, your hand should fall along the back of your hips. Throughout the motion, make sure they swing back and forth in a straight motion that's in sync with your feet. Doing so not only helps you stay balanced (so you don't lose momentum), but it can help you control your walking speed: The quicker you swing your arms, the quicker your pace will pick up when you need to kick it into high gear.

Finally, make sure you pick the right type of shoes to walk in before you take your first step. You don't have to invest in a walking shoe because a pair of good running shoes, cross-trainers, or light trail hiking boots will also work just fine for the monthlong plan. But whatever you wear should have good arch support and an upper made of materials that let your feet breathe (such as leather or nylon mesh).

The Maximum Metabolism Workout: Blast Away Your Belly Fat

SELLING YOU ON THE BENEFITS of building lean muscle shouldn't be that difficult, especially because it's typically on every guy's wish list. After all, who wouldn't want to be—and look—stronger, fitter, and more powerful? But when it comes to muscle, a lot of men haven't the slightest idea why it's so important when it comes to keeping their guts in check. The truth is, the more lean muscle you have, the more calories your body has to burn to maintain every pound. The end result: a metabolism that stays revved at a higher rate, all the time.

The fact is, the more muscle you have, the more fat you'll melt off even when you're standing still, watching the game, or sleeping all night long. There's only one problem: After age 30, your body loses roughly half a pound of muscle per year, which can lead to your body burning up to 15 less calories each day. The numbers get even worse when you hit 40 because your body's metabolism begins to decline at a rate of 3 percent to 5 percent per decade. It's the reason most men have a harder time losing their belly fat as they get older. Even if you're still eating the same amount of calories as you did when you were younger, having less muscle and a slower metabolism leaves your body no choice but to burn fewer calories and store whatever is remaining as unwanted fat.

Doing a weight-training routine can change all that by minimizing muscle loss and giving your metabolism the shot in the arm it needs. All it takes is performing the right full-body workout three times a week to not only preserve the muscle that you already have, but to help build more lean muscle to boost your metabolism even higher.

What makes this routine ideal is that it boosts your metabolism and builds your muscles in a way that's virtually excuse-proof. For Weeks 1 and 2, the workouts are designed so that they take less than 10 minutes to perform. Even though your workouts become more intense for Weeks 3 and 4, you can still do them—from start to finish—in less than 20 minutes max. The secret to shaving time is that each workout is set up as a circuit—with minimal time in between each exercise. By spending fewer seconds resting between moves, you'll push your muscles—and your metabolism—even harder (and see more results) in far less time than the average workout most men tend to stick with.

Muscle Mayhem!

Once your muscles get used to an exercise routine, you'll start to see fewer results and may even stop seeing results altogether (a situation most guys know as "plateauing"). To keep your muscles from adapting, this workout relies on a training method known as "undulating periodization," which changes the reps, sets, and rest periods you use in every single workout. It may seem confusing, but it's a technique that prevents your muscles from adapting too quickly to your workouts, which is why researchers from Arizona State University found it to be one of the most effective ways to increase overall muscle strength.[2]

Before You Start: Weight Lifting Basics

IF YOU'RE PICKING UP DUMBBELLS for the first time, here are some strength-training basics that you'll need to know to get started.

Know the lingo: A *rep* (short for repetition) is simply an exercise performed one time. A *set* is a group of repetitions. For example, doing one set of 10 repetitions means you'll perform the exercise 10 times.

Push yourself appropriately: For each exercise, you want to start with a moderate weight that lets you perform the required number of repetitions. As you get stronger, you'll need to increase the amount of weight you're using to keep your muscles challenged. You can do that by either raising the weight by $2\frac{1}{2}$ to 5 pounds in that particular exercise, or if you like, opt to do the harder version of the exercise.

Don't make the mistake of trying to use too much weight, thinking that you'll see faster results. Choosing a weight that's more than what you should use will only increase your risk of getting injured, which will bring your entire exercise regime to a halt.

If you can't do the recommended number of repetitions, then the weight's too heavy. Lower the weight you're using until you find the right amount. If you can do more repetitions than recommended, then the weight's too light, so increase the weight. Odds are, picking a weight that's too light for you will happen to you on the first try. When researchers at Grand Valley State University asked subjects to pick weights they thought were heavy enough for them to exercise with, all of them chose weights that were lighter than what they should have been using.[3] That's fine, so long as you make sure to adjust accordingly.

Pay attention to the numbers: At the start of this 4-week program, you'll be doing one set of 10, 12, or 15 reps (depending on the day). As you progress, you'll jump up to doing two sets of 10, 12, or 15 reps (again, depending on the day).

Watch the clock: As you progress through the routine, the time you'll rest between each of the four exercises will shrink, By reducing how long you'll linger between sets, you'll transform each workout into a circuit-training routine, a technique that turns your muscle-building routine into a cardiovascular workout simultaneously by also challenging your heart and lungs. As you lift, your weight lifting workout will turn into an aerobic, fat-burning experience. That length of time will range from 60 seconds in between to as little as no rest in between, so follow the instructions to the letter.

Pick the right moves: If you have never done any weight-training exercises (or haven't exercised in more than 6 months) or if you have knee problems, start with the Make It Easier option that's available with each weight-training exercise. Otherwise, start with the Main Move. If that's too challenging, perform the Make It Easier option. If it's not challenging enough, perform the Make It Harder option. The same rule applies to the abdominal exercises in the Cut to the Core Routine.

Maximum Metabolism Workout Weekly Plan

WEEK	DAY 2	DAY 4	DAY 6
1	10 reps (rest 30 seconds between exercises)	15 reps (rest 60 seconds between exercises)	12 reps (rest 45 seconds between exercises)
2	15 reps (rest 45 seconds between exercises)	12 reps (rest 30 seconds between exercises)	10 reps (rest 15 seconds between exercises)
3	2 sets, 12 reps (rest 30 seconds between exercises)	2 sets, 10 reps (rest 15 seconds between exercises)	2 sets, 15 reps (rest 45 seconds between exercises)
4	2 sets, 10 reps (no rest between exercises)	2 sets, 15 reps (rest 30 seconds between exercises)	2 sets, 12 reps (rest 15 seconds between exercises)

Pull in the Right Direction

Keeping your muscles flexible by stretching after your workout (when your muscles are warm and pliable) helps keep your belly flat in several ways. Exercising regularly tightens your ligaments, which can pull your spine out of alignment and lead to poor posture. Stretching loosens your ligaments, making it easier to stand straighter and prevent any slouching from making your belly look bigger than it really is. It can also make your muscles less susceptible to strains and cramps and allow them to recover faster from exercise by flushing out lactic acid. This helps you stay on target to meet all of your exercise goals.

Because most guys hate to stretch, we devised three multimuscle timesaving moves that loosen several muscles at once. Perform each stretch 3 to 6 times to make sure you've worked each area thoroughly before moving on to the next stretch.

STRETCH #1: *(Loosens the shoulders and triceps)*

Raise your arms overhead and hold your right elbow with your left hand. Let your right hand drop down behind your neck. Now gently pull your right elbow to the left and behind your head. Hold for 5 seconds then release. Repeat with the left elbow.

STRETCH #2: *(Loosens the back, buttocks, and legs)*

Lie on your back with both legs flat on the floor. Bend your right knee up and wrap your hands underneath your kneecap. Gently pull your right knee toward your chest as far as is comfortable, keeping your head on the floor as you go, and hold for 3 seconds. Slowly bring the leg back to the floor and repeat with the left leg.

STRETCH #3: *(Loosens the upper back, chest, spine, and waist)*

Stand with your back straight, knees unlocked, and feet wider than shoulder-width apart. Place your left hand flat against the outside of your left thigh and raise your right arm straight over your head, palm facing forward. Begin to exhale as you slowly lean your body to the left, letting your left hand slide down toward your ankle as far as you can. Hold this pose for 10 deep breaths, then bring yourself back up, inhaling as you go. Switch arms, this time placing your right hand on your right leg, raising your left, and repeating the move to the right for 10 more breaths.

Lunging Deadlift

(works the quadriceps, hamstrings, glutes, trapezius, and lower back)

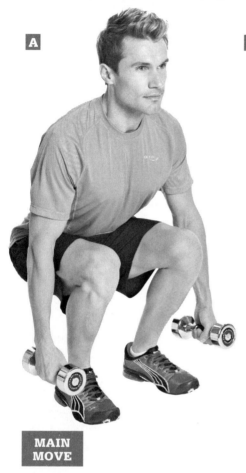

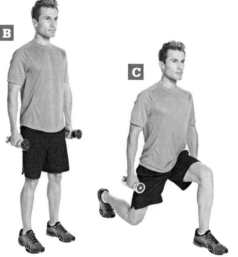

MAIN MOVE

A. Stand with your feet spaced 6 to 8 inches apart with a dumbbell placed along the outside of each foot. Bend your knees and grab the dumbbells so that your palms face in toward each other. Before you begin the exercise, make sure that your back and shoulders are straight (not rounded), and your head is up.

B. Keeping your head and back straight, slowly stand up until your legs are straight—knees unlocked—keeping the dumbbells close to your body as you lift.

C. Keeping your back straight, take a large step forward with your left foot and bend your knees until your left leg forms a 90-degree angle. Your upper left thigh should be almost parallel to the floor. Reverse the motion, lightly pushing off of your left foot, until you're back in a standing position.

D. (not pictured) Once your legs are back together, slowly lower the weights to the floor (but don't let go of them) and repeat, this time, stepping forward with your right foot.

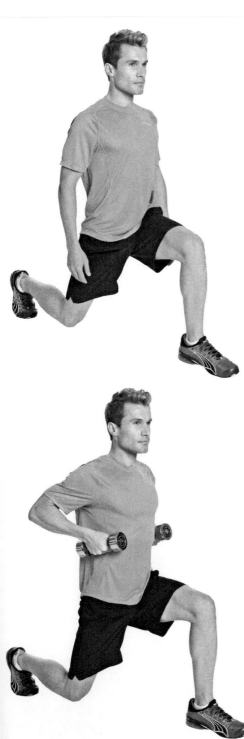

**MAKE IT
EASIER**

Instead of lowering the weights down after each lunge in Step D, do it after every two lunges (after you've stepped forward with both your left and right foot). Or, try doing the whole exercise without weights until you get the hang of the movement.

**MAKE IT
HARDER**

As you step forward in Step C, pull the weights straight up to the edges of your chest (your elbows should flare out to your sides). As you step back into a standing position, lower them back down.

Front Squat Press Curl

(works the quadriceps, hamstrings, glutes, shoulders, biceps, and triceps)

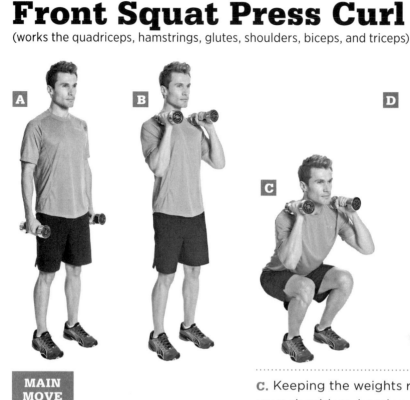

A **B** **C** **D**

MAIN MOVE

A. Stand with a dumbbell in each hand, arms hanging down at your sides with your palms facing in toward the sides of your thighs. Your legs should be straight, knees unlocked.

B. Curl the weights up without rotating your wrists so that the end of each dumbbell rests comfortably on the front of each shoulder.

C. Keeping the weights resting on your shoulders, bend your knees and sit back as if you were going to sit in a chair (your knees should stay behind your toes at all times). Stop when your thighs are parallel to the floor.

D. Push yourself back up into a standing position, then immediately press the weights overhead until your arms are straight, elbows unlocked.

E. (not pictured) Lower the weights back down to your shoulders, then curl them down so that your arms are hanging along your sides. Repeat the exercise for the required number of repetitions.

Instead of squatting all the way down in Step C, only lower yourself about one-quarter or half of the way.

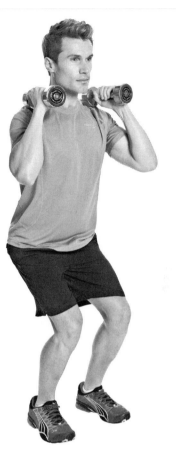

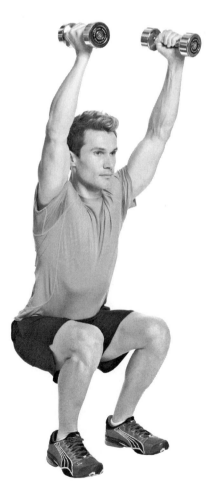

MAKE IT HARDER

Try adding a second squat into the middle of the routine. After you've come to standing with weights pressed overhead in Step D, slowly lower yourself back down into another squat, keeping the weights raised above you as you squat, then stand back up. Afterward, simply lower the weights down to your shoulders, then curl them back down as usual.

Angled Lunge Row

(works the quadriceps, hamstrings, glutes, upper back, and biceps)

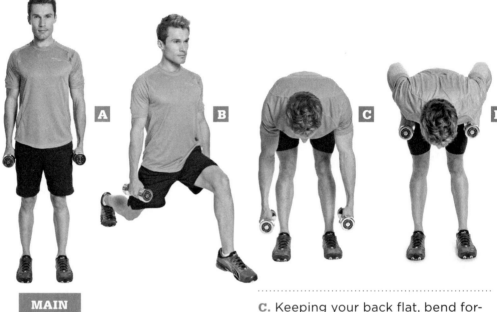

MAIN MOVE

A. Stand holding a dumbbell in each hand with your feet shoulder-width apart. Your arms should hang down at your sides, palms facing in toward each other.

B. Take a big step with your left foot, dropping it slightly forward and out to your side about 2 to 3 feet. (If you were standing in the center of a clock facing 12, your left foot would be between 10 and 11.) Keeping your back straight, slowly bend your left leg until your left thigh is parallel to the floor—your knee should stay behind your toes. Push yourself back up into a standing position.

C. Keeping your back flat, bend forward at your hips until your torso is almost parallel to the floor, letting your arms hang down with your palms facing in.

D. Bend your elbows back and pull the weights straight up until they reach the sides of your chest. Lower the weights back down, then stand up into the start position.

E. (not pictured) Repeat the exercise with the opposite leg, this time by stepping out to the right with your right foot, then bending your right leg until your right thigh is parallel to the floor. That's one rep.

MAKE IT EASIER

(not pictured) Instead of doing a row after every lunge, do it after every two lunges (after you've stepped forward with both your left and right foot).

MAKE IT HARDER

Instead of rowing both weights up together in Step D, raise them one arm at a time to challenge your stability.

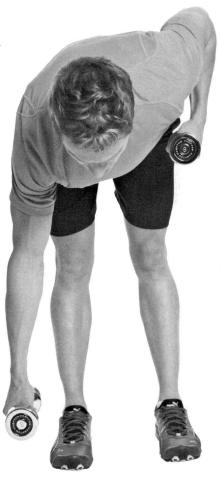

Squat Thrust Push-Up

(works the quadriceps, hamstrings, glutes, chest, shoulders, and triceps)

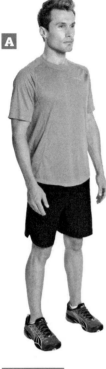

A

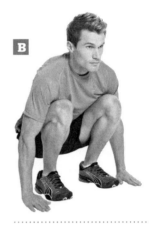

B

B. Quickly squat down as deep as you can and place your hands on the floor, shoulder-width apart.

MAIN MOVE

A. Stand with your feet shoulder-width apart, arms down by your sides.

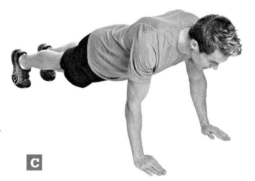

C

C. Keeping your hands on the floor, step your feet out one at a time so that your legs are straight behind you—you should end up in a pushup position. Quickly do one pushup, then step your feet forward to the spot where they were before, and immediately stand up.

Before doing each pushup
in Step C, gently place both
knees on the floor.

**MAKE IT
HARDER**

(not pictured) Once your hands
touch the floor in Step B, quickly
kick your legs out straight behind
you (instead of stepping back with
each leg) to get into a pushup
position. After doing one pushup,
quickly pull your knees back into
your chest, then immediately
stand up.

Cut to the Core Routine

THE THIRD PORTION OF the Flat Belly Workout targets the muscles you're looking to see in the first place: your abdominals. But to make this workout unique and one of the easiest routines you've ever tried, we fused five of the best and most effective ab exercises into one routine that strengthens and shreds all of the core muscles your belly's been hiding all these years. The best part: Each move has been shown to be more effective than doing a traditional crunch, which should explain why you won't be doing a single crunch in the entire 28-day program.

The Toe Reach works the upper portion of your rectus abdominis, which connects from the bottom of your ribs down to your pelvis. It also indirectly strengthens the lower portion of your rectus abdominis, as well as your obliques (the muscles that wrap around your sides). The best part of all: It's a move that's been shown to be 29 percent more effective at activating your rectus abdominus and 116 percent more efficient at activating your obliques than a standard crunch.

The Stability Sit also works your entire rectus abdominus, but in a unique way that trains all of your core muscles at the same time—without having to move a muscle. This balance move keeps your ab muscles continuously contracted so you activate more muscle fibers throughout your midsection.

The Leg Scissor specifically focuses on the lower portion of your rectus abdominus, an area that most men tend to neglect. Targeting this area not only

Don't Hold Your Breath

Don't hold your breath—or breathe too forcefully—as you run through the workout. Instead, just breathe normally during each exercise, inhaling as you lower yourself and exhaling as you raise yourself. In fact, try exhaling as much as you can during the up position. This trick can help contract your abdominal muscles even further.

guarantees that your entire abdominal wall will look great from top to bottom, but it also prevents any weak links between your upper and lower body whenever they work together to transfer energy during any activity.

The Knee Lift and Lower also hits the lower portion of your abs, but its twisting motion focuses on the obliques, generating 140 percent more activity than the traditional crunch. Not only does this type of move shape up your midsection even faster, but it develops functional strength at your core that can help you tap more power when you swing a bat, toss a ball, or throw a punch.

Finally, the Floor Hyperextension doesn't specifically strengthen the abs, but works the lower back muscles behind them, which are an integral part of the muscular structure that makes up your core. By rounding off your routine with this move, you'll tighten your entire waist from front to back, making it easier to maintain perfect posture—and minimize any slouching that can create the illusion of a bigger belly—all day long.

One final tip to jack up results: Breathe in and out as you exercise, but concentrate on pulling in your stomach—as if you were trying to impress someone at the beach by looking slimmer. Sucking in your gut strengthens your transverse abdominus (a thin area of muscle that stretches across your midsection). This little trick done with all five exercises strengthens this muscle to help improve your posture, making your abs look impressively flatter all day long!

Cut to the Core Routine Weekly Plan

WEEK	DAY 2	DAY 4	DAY 6
1	8–10 reps	8–10 reps	8–10 reps
2	12–15 reps	12–15 reps	12–15 reps
3	2 sets, 8–10 reps	2 sets, 8–10 reps	2 sets, 8–10 reps
4	2 sets, 12–15 reps	2 sets, 12–15 reps	2 sets, 12–15 reps

Toe Reach

(works the rectus abdominus and obliques)

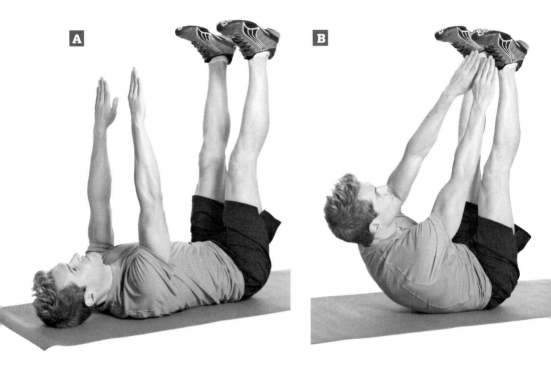

MAIN MOVE

A. Lie flat and raise your arms and legs so your hands and feet point toward the ceiling, spacing your feet shoulder-width apart.

B. Raise up and reach with both hands toward your right foot, lifting your head and shoulders off the floor.

C. (not pictured) Lower yourself back down, then repeat the exercise, this time reaching for your left foot. That's one rep. Continue alternating from right to left, keeping your arms and legs raised during the entire exercise.

Bend your knees and place your feet flat on the floor. Instead of reaching for your feet, imagine you're reaching for the ceiling.

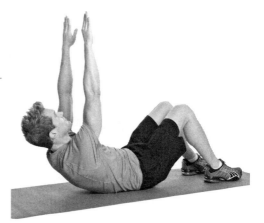

Hold a light medicine ball in your hands throughout the exercise. Instead of reaching with your hands, aim the edge of the ball toward each foot.

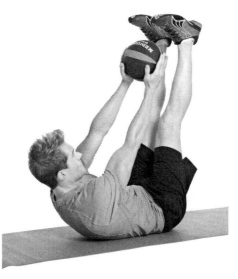

Leg Scissor

(works the lower portion of the rectus abdominus)

A. Lie flat with your legs straight, arms at your sides with your hands tucked underneath your buttocks, palms down. Keeping your legs straight and together, raise them up a few feet so that they are around a 45-degree angle.

A

B. Holding this posture, slowly cross your right foot over your left foot.

C. (not pictured) Pause, then separate your feet about shoulder-width apart and recross them, this time placing your left foot over your right foot. That's one rep. Repeat the exercise for the required repetitions.

B

**MAKE IT
EASIER**

Instead of lying flat, sit on the
floor, extend your arms behind
you, and place your hands flat
on the floor. Lean back
so that your arms support
your weight, then raise
your legs off the floor
and begin crossing your
feet over each other.

**MAKE IT
HARDER**

Lower your legs so that your feet are
closer to the floor. The lower to the
floor they are, the more difficult the
exercise will feel.

Stability Sit
(works the entire rectus abdominus)

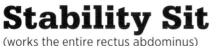

A. Sit on the floor, legs bent, knees together, and feet flat. Reach your arms forward so they touch the outside of your knees, palms facing down.

B. Keeping your legs fixed in a bent position, slowly lean back, raising your feet a few inches off the ground. Ideally, you want your torso and thighs to be at a 45-degree angle so that you're shaped like the letter V.

C. (not pictured) Balance in this position for 6 to 8 seconds, then lean forward and place your feet back on the floor for a 1- to 2-second rest. Repeat the exercise for the required repetitions.

Instead of raising your feet off the floor, keep them flat on the floor through the entire exercise. Then lean back 45 degrees and hold yourself in this position for as long as you can for up to 6 to 8 seconds.

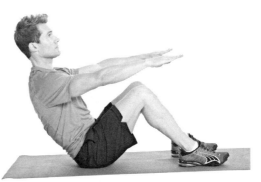

As you balance yourself in Step B, slowly twist your torso to the left for 2 to 3 seconds, return to center, then twist to the right for 2 to 3 seconds.

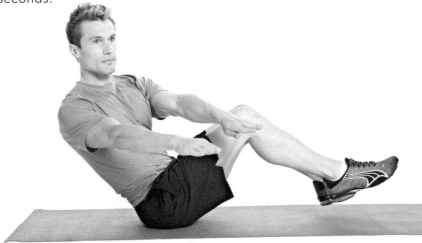

Knee Lift and Lower

(works the lower portion of the rectus abdominus and obliques)

MAIN MOVE

A. Lie flat with your arms extended out to your sides, palms facing down. Your legs should be straight, knees unlocked, and flat on the floor.

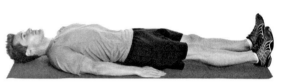

B. This move breaks down into three parts. (1) Keeping your heels on the floor, bend your knees and pull your feet toward your butt. (2) Lift your feet off the floor as you pull your knees up toward your chest as far as you comfortably can. (3) Raise your hips off the floor, then twist your knees to the right. Try to keep your back and butt in contact as much as possible with the floor.

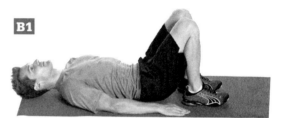

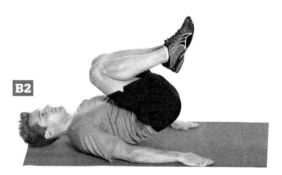

C. (not pictured) Reverse the motion by slowly twisting your knees back above your chest, lowering your feet to the floor by your butt, then straightening your legs.

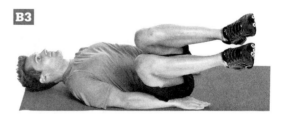

D. (not pictured) Repeat the exercise, this time drawing your knees up, then dropping them to your left side.

MAKE IT EASIER

Instead of twisting your knees side to side at the top, just draw your knees up to your chest, then lower them back down to the floor.

MAKE IT HARDER

Keep your heels raised about an inch above the floor for the entire exercise.

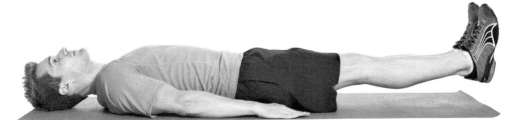

Floor Hyperextension

(works the lower back)

A. Lie facedown on your stomach on a mat, arms extended so that your upper arms are by your ears. Your legs should be extended straight behind you.

B. Slowly lift your chest and arms off the floor as high as you comfortably can, keeping your arms straight and in line with your torso as you go—your feet and legs should stay on the ground. Pause at the top for 1 second, then lower yourself back to the floor. Repeat the exercise for the required repetitions.

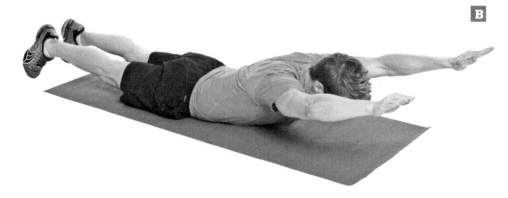

MAKE IT EASIER

Instead of extending your arms in front of you in Step A, bend your arms, place your hands on top of one another on the floor, then rest your forehead on them. As you lift your chest off the floor in Step B, keep your arms bent as you raise them with your torso.

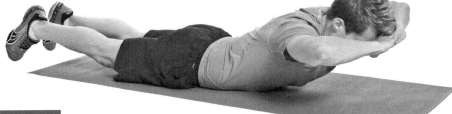

MAKE IT HARDER

As you raise your torso off the floor in Step B, raise your legs at the same time.

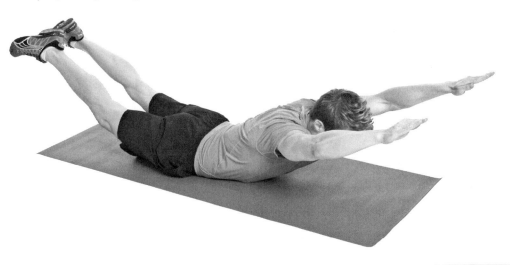

YOUR 28-DAY FLAT BELLY DIET FOR MEN WORKOUT PLAN

WEEK	DAY 1	DAY 2	DAY 3	
1	FAT BLAST WALK 30 minutes CUT TO THE CORE ROUTINE 8–10 reps	CALORIE TORCH WALK 25 minutes MAXIMUM METABOLISM WORKOUT 10 reps	FAT BLAST WALK 30 minutes CUT TO THE CORE ROUTINE 8–10 reps	
2	FAT BLAST WALK 45 minutes CUT TO THE CORE ROUTINE 12–15 reps	CALORIE TORCH WALK 35 minutes MAXIMUM METABOLISM WORKOUT 15 reps	FAT BLAST WALK 45 minutes CUT TO THE CORE ROUTINE 12–15 reps	
3	FAT BLAST WALK 60 minutes CUT TO THE CORE ROUTINE 2 sets, 8–10 reps	CALORIE TORCH WALK 45 minutes MAXIMUM METABOLISM WORKOUT 2 sets, 12 reps	FAT BLAST WALK 60 minutes CUT TO THE CORE ROUTINE 2 sets, 8–10 reps	
4	FAT BLAST WALK 60 minutes CUT TO THE CORE ROUTINE 2 sets, 12–15 reps	CALORIE TORCH WALK 45 minutes MAXIMUM METABOLISM WORKOUT 2 sets, 10 reps	FAT BLAST WALK 60 minutes CUT TO THE CORE ROUTINE 2 sets, 12–15 reps	

DAY 4	DAY 5	DAY 6	DAY 7
CALORIE TORCH WALK 25 minutes	FAT BLAST WALK 30 minutes	CALORIE TORCH WALK 25 minutes	REST
MAXIMUM METABOLISM WORKOUT 15 reps	CUT TO THE CORE ROUTINE 8–10 reps	MAXIMUM METABOLISM WORKOUT 12 reps	
CALORIE TORCH WALK 35 minutes	FAT BLAST WALK 45 minutes	CALORIE TORCH WALK 35 minutes	REST
MAXIMUM METABOLISM WORKOUT 12 reps	CUT TO THE CORE ROUTINE 12–15 reps	MAXIMUM METABOLISM WORKOUT 10 reps	
CALORIE TORCH WALK 45 minutes	FAT BLAST WALK 60 minutes	CALORIE TORCH WALK 45 minutes	REST
MAXIMUM METABOLISM WORKOUT 2 sets, 8–10 reps	CUT TO THE CORE ROUTINE 2 sets, 8–10 reps	MAXIMUM METABOLISM WORKOUT 2 sets, 15 reps	
CALORIE TORCH WALK 45 minutes	FAT BLAST WALK 60 minutes	CALORIE TORCH WALK 45 minutes	REST
MAXIMUM METABOLISM WORKOUT 2 sets, 15 reps	CUT TO THE CORE ROUTINE 2 sets, 12–15 reps	MAXIMUM METABOLISM WORKOUT 2 sets, 12 reps	

YOU ASK, WE ANSWER

BEFORE YOU GET STARTED, here are some of the questions our test panelists asked. Knowing the answers ahead of time will give you an edge to extra weight loss by helping you achieve even better results!

Q Is it OK to eat right before I exercise if I'm hungry? Many guys believe that exercising on an empty stomach burns more fat. Not true. The fact is, having a preworkout snack that's a mix of carbohydrates and protein within 2 hours of exercising is entirely OK, especially if you run the risk of feeling less energized to really push yourself through your workouts. Some smart, less-filling choices include: a cup of plain low-fat yogurt with a tablespoon of raisins or walnuts or a slice of whole wheat bread with a tablespoon of peanut butter and jelly and a glass of fat-free milk.

Q What should I be drinking as I exercise? Staying hydrated before, during, and after exercise is crucial if you're serious about losing weight, especially since dehydration can minimize your strength, sap your energy levels, and leave you less likely to finish your workout. But what's the best formula to follow when working out? Start hydrating 15 to 30 minutes before you exercise by drinking at least 16 to 32 ounces of water. Then, try to drink at least 8 to 12 ounces of water every 15 minutes as you work out. Best bet: Choose regular (and calorie-less) water over sports drinks, which are really only necessary if you plan on exercising over an hour.

Q What if I want to do my workouts on a treadmill instead of walking outside? That's fine. It doesn't matter where you walk, as long as you make the right adjustments. When you walk outside, you're the one moving yourself forward. Because a treadmill rotates the surface for you, it reduces how hard you work. However, that's easy to fix. Just raise the treadmill to a 1 percent incline—this adds just the right amount of extra resistance to your routines so that your body, heart, and lungs work just as hard as they would walking on a flat surface outside.

Q Should I use a weight belt when lifting? Guys love weight belts, but unless you've recently suffered a back injury or are doing Olympic-level exercises (none of which you'll find in this book), it's not necessary to use one. In fact, it could prevent your midsection from becoming as strong as it could be. That's because wearing a belt creates external pressure that helps your abdominal muscles support your spine and lower back, instead of allowing your muscles to learn how to do the job themselves. Using a belt too often can prevent the muscles within your torso from getting any stronger, which could make them more susceptible to injury when you're not wearing one doing ordinary lifting. Instead, lightly tighten your midsection as you begin each set. Keeping your ab muscles contracted throughout each exercise should allow your transverse abdominus to help you maintain your posture perfectly.

 Q I have trouble staying committed to an exercise program. Do you have any tips? Staying the course can be tough, but there are two tricks you can try that work for a lot of men. (1) Treat every workout as if it was an important business meeting, then write it down into your daily planner before anything else you have to do that day. After that, work the rest of your schedule around it. (2) Find someone

to exercise with. Going through the Flat Belly Diet for Men routines with a workout partner won't just help you push yourself harder, but it will make you accountable to someone else (so you'll be less likely to blow off a workout on days when you feel less motivated).

Q Is there anything else I could be doing to help my muscles grow? Thanks to this chapter, you already have all the fitness tools you need to achieve your muscle-building (and weight loss) goals. However, the single biggest factor most men never take as seriously as their workouts is sleep. You already know how catching enough Z's can affect your metabolism, but it's equally important to help your muscles rebuild themselves so they can become stronger and fitter. If you don't give your body enough sleep, your muscles never get the chance to improve, which can stall your progress (no matter how much hard work you've put in). To keep your muscles growing so they can help burn off more fat, make sure you're allowing yourself at least 8 hours of sleep each night.

Staying the Course

THERE ARE A LOT OF TRICKS you can use to help keep yourself motivated and reap even more benefits throughout the entire 28-day program. We'll give you four right now:

1. WEAR HEADPHONES. Listening to tunes while exercising doesn't just keep your mind from being bored, it can help your body burn more calories. Researchers at Ohio State University found that subjects who listened to music while walking felt physically less exhausted and walked an average of 21 percent farther than usual. Subjects without tunes actually walked an average of 169 feet less.[4]

2. TURN OFF THE TV. A study performed by Harvard researchers found that subjects walked 144 steps less each day for every hour of TV they watched. By shaving an hour off your nightly TV schedule, you'll end up strengthening your heart and muscles by walking an extra 2 miles a month without even realizing it.[5]

3. WEAR WHAT YOU LIKE. According to researchers at the University of Wisconsin, dressing in exercise clothes you feel comfortable in can help you lose more weight. Their research found that subjects who wore more casual clothing

Walk to Lose for the Long Haul

It may not feel as intense as running, but research has shown that walking may be the key to taking off—and keeping off—excess body fat. A 4-year study funded by the National Institutes of Health found that subjects who participated in "lifestyle activities" totaling at least 30 minutes of moderate-intensity physical activity each day—such as walking—lost as much weight and made greater gains in fitness than participants who did aerobic exercise 4 days a week for 40 minutes a session. Subjects who walked were also more likely to maintain their fitness improvements a year later.[8]

Weights Whittle Fat

If you think that only cardio training burns calories, you're wrong. According to research performed at the Department of Exercise, Sport and Health Studies at the University of Texas at Arlington, men burn an average of 6.2 calories a minute during a free-weight circuit routine (just like the one recommended in this program).[6]

at work took an average of 491 extra steps a day, burning close to 8 percent more calories compared to subjects who were more burdened by the clothes they wore when exercising.[7]

4. DON'T OVERDO IT. The workouts in this book get results because they use exercises and routines that are just the right intensity. However, listen to your body. Overdoing it by pushing yourself harder than you feel comfortable with or ignoring any pain you may be experiencing only increases your chances of getting sidelined with an injury. That also goes for trying to do activities in addition to the program, such as other exercise routines, sports, or anything that may prevent your body from getting the rest it needs between workouts. Instead, your safest bet is sticking with the 28-day plan, then using the rest of your time to rest and focus on your diet.

As easy as these tips may be for keeping you on track, the biggest tool you can turn to is your brain. It may sound crazy, but believing that you can stick with the entire program is truly the key to making sure you will. Don't believe your mind has a lot to do with your body? In a Harvard study, subjects who believed they were getting a good workout showed greater reductions in fat loss and blood pressure than subjects who performed the same activities but didn't feel they were exercising.[9] That means that simply convincing yourself that you're burning more fat as you exercise can make it happen. It also means that if you decide to stay on track, you will stay on track—so take advantage of it!

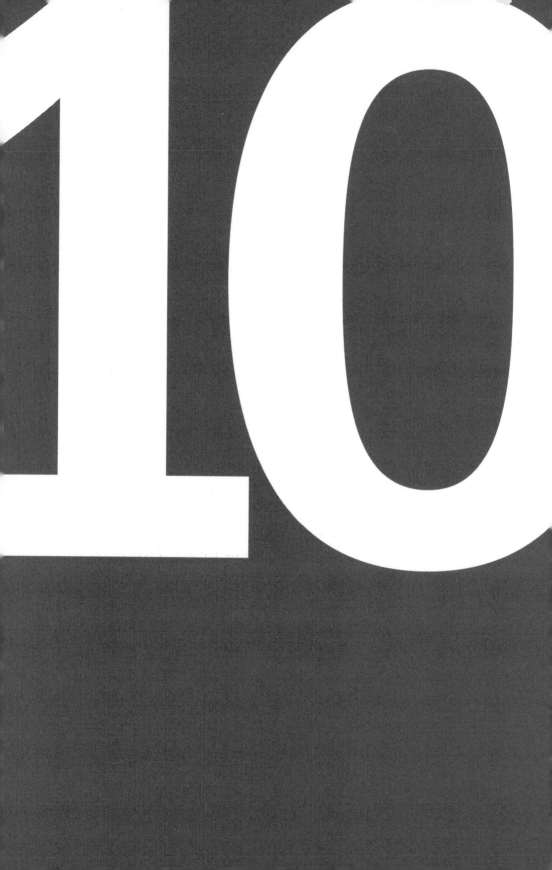

YOUR GUIDE TO DAY 33 AND BEYOND

CONGRATULATIONS, YOU'VE NOW finished the full 32 days of the Flat Belly Diet for Men. You should be proud of yourself—and your shrunken gut—for coming this far. But your work doesn't end here if you want to permanently keep that spare tire off. Doing a diet in a vacuum won't help you in the long run. The healthy habits you've acquired through this program have to become part of your lifestyle.

The good news is that more and more people in the United States are turning to a healthier lifestyle. One study shows that 57 percent of grocery shoppers are trying to eat healthfully, up from 45 percent in 2000.[1] Americans are eating more fruits, veggies, and whole grains, and in some surveys as many as 90 percent are doing something to improve the healthfulness of their meals, like limiting salt, sugar, or saturated fat or paying more attention to portions. What does this all mean? To me it implies that we're now more interested in making food choices that impact our long-term health rather than turning to fad, quick-fix plans. That's why I wanted the Flat Belly Diet for Men to be, first and foremost, something you guys could sustain for the rest of your lives.

Taking a Look Back

BEFORE WE GET INTO how you're going to maintain your smaller gut—and better health—let's take a look at how far you've come. You've learned a few things about how your body works and the mind's impact on your physical health. You know, for instance, the toll that stress can take on a guy, as well as why the fat you can't see is sometimes scarier than the stuff hanging over your pants. And if you've followed the parameters of this plan (eating your MUFAs at every meal, limiting calories to 2,000 a day, exercising regularly, and approaching food in a healthy way), then you've already taken the most difficult step toward a healthier future. You should have also lost some of the deadliest fat out there in the process: belly fat.

I hope that after completing the 32-day plan and sticking to its simple rules, you've realized that you want to continue with this diet for the long run. Our test panelists certainly did. After ending the test phase of the Flat Belly Diet for Men, every single guy said he planned to stick with the program. Why? Because they'd lost weight and inches, including around the waist. The men were also able to maintain high energy levels, never felt starved, and loved the food on the diet—whether they were following the quick-fix meals or the recipes. In fact, most of them said they didn't even feel like they were on a diet the whole time. Hopefully this rings true for you, too! Succeeding on the Flat Belly Diet for Men is ultimately about more than just losing your paunch: It promises a longer, healthier life.

This chapter is about getting you fully armed to reap all the rewards of the Flat Belly Diet for Men—shrunken gut included—for decades to come. The first step is to permanently adopt the three rules, which you're probably quite familiar with by now.

Flat Belly for Life: The Three Flat Belly Diet for Men Rules

- **RULE #1:** Stick to 400 calories per meal.
- **RULE #2:** Never go more than 4 hours without eating.
- **RULE #3:** Eat a MUFA at every meal.

Rule #1: Stick to 400 Calories per Meal

YOU MUST CONTINUE to control your daily caloric intake to keep your weight down and your metabolism on track. This means sticking to about 400 calories per meal, 2,000 calories per day—even if you've reached your weight loss goals. The reality is that 2,000 calories is enough to keep your energy levels up, support your immune system, and maintain your calorie-burning muscle (so you don't feel tired, cranky, or hungry), but it's not enough calories to allow your gut to return. If you're starting to envision a life of potential deprivation or boredom, remember this: You've been on the Flat Belly Diet for Men for 32 days now and know firsthand how satisfying it is. Between the quick-fix meals, Power Snacks, recipes, and multitude of approved packaged and fast-food items, there's no time to feel bored or deprived on this eating plan. You have hundreds of food choices, whether or not you have the time (or the inclination) to cook.

Rule #2: Never Go More Than 4 Hours without Eating

IF YOU'VE BEEN FOLLOWING this rule consistently, then you should have established an eating rhythm by now. In response, your body will be used to having three MUFA-rich 400-calorie meals at 4-hour intervals, as well as two healthy Power Snacks at whatever time of day suits you. This eating schedule should have helped maintain your energy levels, revved your metabolism, and stabilized your blood sugar. In other words, you now have control of your appetite. Stick with this schedule and it will continue to benefit your health and your waistline.

Rule #3: Eat a MUFA at Every Meal

BY NOW YOU SHOULD BE very familiar with the various MUFAs. These super-nutrients—found mainly in vegetable oils, nuts, seeds, olives, and avocados—help you feel full and lose visceral fat from your middle. You've likely also discovered how easy it is to include small amounts of these healthy fats in all your meals and snacks. So continue with the MUFA habit going forward, and your belly will thank you. Don't stress if you can't work in a MUFA at every single meal and snack—just do the best you can. If you don't know the MUFA list by heart at this point, you can always flip to page 99 for a quick reference.

Six Sustainable Strategies

This diet isn't just about rules, though; it's really about your attitude. The same rings true for this eating plan going forward. You have all the tools and tricks you need to get rid of your spare tire and maintain a healthy life. This toolbox of strategies is just as important for your continued success as the MUFAs and the meals as you go past Day 32 of the Flat Belly Diet for Men.

Use the following key practices and pointers as a guide for your future on this plan:

Control Stress

The stress/belly fat connection is clear. If you manage your stress levels, you are one step closer to permanently managing your belly fat. Hanging out with your buddies can be a great stress reliever, as can going for a walk or a jog. Every guy has his own ways of dealing with stress, but the main thing is that you're doing something to keep anxiety levels low. Don't forget to revisit Chapter 4 if you need more ideas to help get your stress under control.

Be Active

Regular activity not only helps reduce stress, it will also ward off your gut for life. Making a habit of combining this eating plan with physical activity will ensure that you'll be healthier overall, and it's also the only way to get those six-pack abs. Be sure to do a mix of cardio, strength training, and core-focused exercises to maximize your workout routine. And remember, stick to activities that you actually enjoy and can do. Feel free to continue following the workout outlined for you in Chapter 9 if it's been working for you so far.

Form a Support Team

You've come this far, so clearly you're motivated and very capable. But still, long-term success is always easier when you have the backing of others. One of the best ways to stay on track and maintain your motivation is to have a support team. Even one buddy or family member will do—just someone to give you that extra boost once in a while. Your supporters don't even have to be members of your family or good friends, as long as they respect your goals and can help keep you focused.

Avoid Weight Gain Traps

Certain scenarios tend to be more gut-inducing than others. For many men, guys' night out, sporting events, and even business travel can lead to more weight gain—in your belly and the rest of your body. While it's unlikely that you can avoid these situations altogether, there are strategies you can use to minimize their impact on your belly. Don't forget to continue using the tips and tricks you've learned to deal with these situations, such as carrying MUFA-rich snacks with you and fitting in exercise wherever you can. Revisit Chapter 4 if you need a reminder of how to deal with these weight loss challenges.

Keep Plateau Perspective

Here's why every dieter hits a weight loss plateau at some point: The Flat Belly Diet for Men is designed to only give you enough calories—2,000—to support a healthy "ideal" weight. By going on this plan, you've created a calorie deficit that will allow you to drop pounds. With every pound you lose, though, this calorie deficit shrinks, so as you get closer and closer to your weight goal, it takes longer and longer to lose the next pound. At times it might feel like your weight loss has stalled. It won't actually be stalled, though perhaps it has slowed. Think of it this way: If you go from losing 2 pounds a week to ¼ pound a week, a loss is still a loss, even if the incremental changes don't register on the scale. Even ¼ pound of fat loss is a full stick of butter zapped from your body, which is amazing progress for 1 week's time!

A good way to stay motivated and avoid the dreaded plateau is to track your progress. Studies show that people who write down what they eat and when they exercise lose more weight than people who don't. We've included a log template for you in the appendix.

A Flat Belly Dining Out Guide

As LONG AS YOU'RE PREPARING your own food, it's simple to follow this eating plan. But what happens when you have a craving to eat out? Or if an anniversary, your buddy's birthday, or some other cause for celebration involves going to a restaurant? We've already been through scenarios that commonly pose weight loss challenges for men, such as guys' night out and sporting events, but unfortunately the eating out challenges don't end there.

Avoiding restaurants isn't a likely solution, but other strategies can help you when you're dining out in the future. The main thing to remember when you eat out is that you're there to socialize, not overeat. If you plan ahead, there's no reason why you can't enjoy a meal anywhere you want, whether it's pizza with the guys or a romantic dinner with your lady. In addition to the tips provided in Chapter 4, follow these guidelines to help you stay on track.

■ Eat what you would normally eat throughout the day. Skipping a meal to save calories for later just increases the chances that you will overeat at dinner. You can also up your exercise—the added calories burned during the activity will help offset a splurge like an appetizer.

■ Have a light snack before you go out. Good options include the pesto turkey rollup, open-faced peanut butter with honey sandwich, a bowl of cereal with fat-free milk and walnuts, or anything that includes a MUFA. The MUFA will take the edge off your hunger and help you pass on the bread basket, nachos, and other pre-meal freebies.

■ Choose the restaurant if possible. This will allow you to research in advance and figure out which places have the best meal options for you. Many restaurants offer their menus online. If not, call ahead so you know what to anticipate menu-wise.

■ Don't hesitate to make special requests or to ask for substitutions to your meal. For instance, get a double order of veggies instead of French fries. If they won't make a substitution, just ask that the belly-inducing food not be included in your meal.

■ Ask to get sauces and dressings on the side if possible. This will allow you to control how much you use on your food and avoid a situation where your meal is slathered with a sauce or dressing.

■ If you can't resist getting an appetizer or dessert, be sure to share it with your dining companion. Often you only need a small amount to satisfy your cravings.

■ Try to leave some food on your plate. Forget what your mom said about cleaning your plate—that rule no longer applies.

Portion Patrol

THE MOST IMPORTANT TIP for dining out is to watch the size of your portions. It goes without saying that anything called "super size" should be avoided, but also be wary of dishes that don't advertise their huge proportions but are actually big enough for two or three people. In fact, many restaurants serve portions that are much bigger than a single serving.

To understand how big is too big when dining out, it helps to have a visual reference of what a serving should look like. For example:

One-half cup of cooked rice or pasta is considered one serving. This is about the size of half a baseball. If you're trying to limit your portion of rice or pasta to two servings, think of one baseball. Most Chinese restaurants provide far more than this amount of rice, and Italian restaurants give you way more pasta than this. Fill up on side orders of steamed veggies.

One standard-size slice of bread is considered one serving of bread. Compare rolls, buns, and other bread products to this mental image and adjust your portion size accordingly. If the bun on your burger looks larger than two slices of bread, for instance, leave some of it on the plate.

Three ounces of cooked meat, the size of a deck of cards, is considered one serving. Most restaurants provide far more than this amount in an entrée. We know you can eat that 18-ounce rib-eye steak—but that doesn't mean that you should. Easy ways to cut back on meat servings include ordering a half portion, having a sandwich instead of an entrée, or splitting a meal.

One-fourth cup of shredded cheese is considered a single portion. That's about the size of a golf ball. According to the 2005 Dietary Guidelines, healthy adults need two to three servings of milk, yogurt, or cheese per day. If cheese is your weakness, think "golf ball" the next time you sprinkle cheese on your food.

A Final Word

WHY ARE YOU doing this diet? Remember that it's for you—your health and your gut. In today's day and age, it's easy to get distracted by all our responsibilities—be it at work or with friends and family—and put our health on the back burner. But we'll pay the price for this later. This is why the Flat Belly Diet for Men was created to be simple and sustainable. It is a weight loss plan based on the most credible—and safe—science that targets the most dangerous type of fat you carry on your body. If you want to live longer and healthier, keeping that belly fat is simply not an option.

I hope that you continue to follow this eating plan and lifestyle for as long as it takes to obtain the freedom that comes from a healthier body weight. And if you end up with six-pack abs, even better! But really, as you know by now, this plan is less about achieving a ripped body than it is about creating a healthier life. If you remember nothing about the Flat Belly Diet for Men except that a MUFA at every meal could save your life, you're still on your way to maximizing your health. My job is now done here. It's time for you to continue the great work you've already started. Good luck!

stats

Food & Exercise Log

IF YOU PLAY OR WATCH SPORTS, you know how important it is to track each players' stats—how far they throw, how high they jump, how fast they run. How else would you know how well your team's doing?

Similarly, it's important for you to track your stats as you aim for your weight loss goal. Writing down what you eat will keep you honest about portion sizes. Observing how hungry you are when you eat can help you identify patterns that may be sabotaging your weight loss. Recording how long or how intense your exercise sessions have been may inspire you to train even more. You don't have to spend hours reflecting on your feelings about your food, just take a few minutes each day to jot down your food intake and activity levels. We've given you a couple of blank food and exercise log pages here to help you get started; photocopy them so that you can take one with you. Alternatively, if you prefer a digital log, check out My Health Trackers at Prevention.com.

Keep the following in mind when filling out your log:

▒ Fill in the **Day** of week and date at the top.

▒ Enter your **Body weight**. Try to weigh yourself at the same time every day, and use the same scale.

▒ In the Food Log, enter your food intake and amounts in the **Food Intake** column. Please be as specific as possible. Make note of the **MUFA** and the total calories in each meal.

▒ Enter the **Time** you ate.

▒ Enter the **Location** at which you ate; please be as specific as possible (i.e., "at home at kitchen table" vs. just "at home").

■ Enter a number under the **Hunger Rating** when starting meal column and **Fullness Rating** when ending meal column using the following scale:

1 = starving, shaky, about to pass out. You want to devour the first thing you see and have a hard time slowing down.

3 = mild to moderate hunger. You have physical symptoms of hunger like a growling tummy and that "I need to eat soon" feeling, but you aren't starving or experiencing any unpleasant symptoms such as a headache, shaking, etc.

5 = just right. My hunger is gone and I feel full but not too full and satisfied. My mind is off food and I'm ready to take on the next task. I feel energized.

8 = a little too much. I think I overdid it. My tummy feels stretched and uncomfortable. I feel kind of sluggish. I may feel satisfied and in a lull. I don't feel energized at all.

10 = way too much. Time to unbutton my pants, curl up in a ball, and wait for the pressure to go away. I definitely overate and feel very uncomfortable.

■ Enter your **Observations** about food in the final column. See the sample we've included for examples.

■ In the Exercise Log, enter which type of **Cardio Exercise** you did (Fat Blast Walk or Calorie Torch Walk) and the **Number of Minutes** you walked. If you didn't do any that day, write "none."

■ Enter which type of **Strength Training** exercise you did and the **Number of Reps** you did, the time of the **Rest** between exercises, and the amount of **Weight Used**. If you didn't do any that day, write "none."

■ Enter your **Observations** about exercise in the final column. See the sample we've included for examples.

SAMPLE FOOD & EXERCISE LOG

DAY/DATE: Week 2, Day 3/Saturday, July 11   BODY WEIGHT: 189

FOOD LOG:

Meal Type	Food Intake	Time	Location	Observations
BREAKFAST Hunger rating when starting meal 3 Fullness rating when ending meal 7	1 cup Kellogg's Cornflakes (100) ½ cup skim milk (45) 2 tbsp pecans (90) ¼ cup raisins (123) ½ medium banana (53) MUFA: pecan Calories: 411	7 am	At kitchen counter, watching morning news while getting ready for work	
LUNCH Hunger rating when starting meal 2 Fullness rating when ending meal 5	Hearty Cobb Salad (from Ch 7) MUFA: avocado Calories: 439	1 pm	In living room, watching the game	Took longer than expected to make salad.
DINNER Hunger rating when starting meal 3 Fullness rating when ending meal 6	Grilled Flank Steak with Olive Oil Mojo Sauce meal (from Ch 8) MUFA: olive oil Calories: 378	8 pm	At kitchen table, sitting down with the wife for a change	
SNACK Hunger rating when starting meal 1 Fullness rating when ending meal 9	1 medium apple (77) with 2 tbsp peanut butter (188) and 1 string cheese (80) and ½ cup popcorn (50) MUFA: peanut butter Calories: 375	5 pm	In kitchen, after mowing the lawn	Starving after mowing lawn. Really wanted a cold beer but settled for Firewater and peanut butter.
SNACK Hunger rating when starting meal 4 Fullness rating when ending meal 8	S'mores (from Ch 7) MUFA: chocolate Calories: 622.5	10 pm	Watching TV	One serving just didn't cut it; had 1 ½.

EXERCISE LOG:

Cardio Exercise	# of Minutes	Strength Training	# of Reps	Rest	Weight Used	Observations
Fat Blast Walk	25 min in morning; 20 min with wife after dinner	Lunging Deadlift Front Squat Press Curl Angled Lunge Row Squat Thrust Pushups (Make It Easier Option)	12 12 12 11	30 sec 30 sec 1 min 1 min	15 lbs 12 lbs 12 lbs	Needed a break by the middle of the circuit, and just couldn't get to the last pushup, even though I went to the easier option after just a couple reps.

FOOD & EXERCISE LOG

DAY/DATE: _____   BODY WEIGHT: _____

FOOD LOG:

Meal Type	Food Intake	Time	Location	Observations
BREAKFAST Hunger rating when starting meal Fullness rating when ending meal				
LUNCH Hunger rating when starting meal Fullness rating when ending meal				
DINNER Hunger rating when starting meal Fullness rating when ending meal				
SNACK Hunger rating when starting meal Fullness rating when ending meal				
SNACK Hunger rating when starting meal Fullness rating when ending meal				

EXERCISE LOG:

Cardio Exercise	# of Minutes	Strength Training	# of Reps	Rest	Weight Used	Observations

FOOD & EXERCISE LOG

DAY/DATE: _____   BODY WEIGHT: _____

FOOD LOG:

Meal Type	Food Intake	Time	Location	Observations
BREAKFAST Hunger rating when starting meal Fullness rating when ending meal				
LUNCH Hunger rating when starting meal Fullness rating when ending meal				
DINNER Hunger rating when starting meal Fullness rating when ending meal				
SNACK Hunger rating when starting meal Fullness rating when ending meal				
SNACK Hunger rating when starting meal Fullness rating when ending meal				

EXERCISE LOG:

Cardio Exercise	# of Minutes	Strength Training	# of Reps	Rest	Weight Used	Observations

FOOD & EXERCISE LOG

DAY/DATE: BODY WEIGHT:

FOOD LOG:

Meal Type	Food Intake	Time	Location	Observations
BREAKFAST Hunger rating when starting meal Fullness rating when ending meal				
LUNCH Hunger rating when starting meal Fullness rating when ending meal				
DINNER Hunger rating when starting meal Fullness rating when ending meal				
SNACK Hunger rating when starting meal Fullness rating when ending meal				
SNACK Hunger rating when starting meal Fullness rating when ending meal				

EXERCISE LOG:

Cardio Exercise	# of Minutes	Strength Training	# of Reps	Rest	Weight Used	Observations

FOOD & EXERCISE LOG

DAY/DATE: _____ BODY WEIGHT: _____

FOOD LOG:

Meal Type	Food Intake	Time	Location	Observations
BREAKFAST Hunger rating when starting meal ___ Fullness rating when ending meal ___				
LUNCH Hunger rating when starting meal ___ Fullness rating when ending meal ___				
DINNER Hunger rating when starting meal ___ Fullness rating when ending meal ___				
SNACK Hunger rating when starting meal ___ Fullness rating when ending meal ___				
SNACK Hunger rating when starting meal ___ Fullness rating when ending meal ___				

EXERCISE LOG:

Cardio Exercise	# of Minutes	Strength Training	# of Reps	Rest	Weight Used	Observations

endnotes

Chapter 1

1. Mayo Clinic staff, MayoClinic.com, Men's Health, "Belly Fat in Men: Why Weight Loss Matters," updated June 23, 2009, http://www.mayoclinic.com/health/belly-fat/MC00054.
2. Weight-control Information Network, National Institute of Diabetes and Digestive and Kidney Diseases, "Statistics Related to Overweight and Obesity," updated May 2007, http://win.niddk.nih.gov/statistics.
3. J. A. Paniagua, A. Gallego de la Sacristana, I. Romero, A. Vidal-Puig, J. M. Latre, E. Sanchez, P. Perez-Martinez, J. Lopez-Miranda, and F. Perez-Jimenez, "Monounsaturated Fat-Rich Diet Prevents Central Body Fat Distribution and Decreases Postprandial Adiponectin Expression Induced by a Carbohydrate-Rich Diet in Insulin-Resistant Subjects," Diabetes Care 3, no. 7 (2007): 1717–23.

Chapter 2

1. Weight-control Information Network, National Institute of Diabetes and Digestive and Kidney Diseases (NIDDK), "Weight and Waist Measurement: Tools for Adults," November 2008, http://win.niddk.nih.gov/publications/tools.htm#circumf.
2. Centers for Disease Control and Prevention, "Heart Disease Is the Number One Cause of Death," February 2, 2009, http://www.cdc.gov/features/heartmonth.
3. American Diabetes Association, "Total Prevalence of Diabetes & Pre-Diabetes," http://www.diabetes.org/diabetes-statistics/prevalence.jsp.
4. Mayo Clinic staff, MayoClinic.com, "Belly Fat in Men: Why Weight Loss Matters," updated June 23, 2009, http://www.mayoclinic.com/health/belly-fat/MC00054.
5. K. Blouin, A. Boivin, and A. Tchernof, "Androgens and Body Fat Distribution," The Journal of Steroid Biochemistry and Molecular Biology 108, nos. 3–5 (2008): 272–80.
6. Harvey B. Simon, The Harvard Medical School Guide to Men's Health: Lessons from the Harvard Men's Health Studies (New York: Free Press, 2004).
7. A. Morrison and J. E. Hokanson, "The Independent Relationship between Triglycerides and Coronary Heart Disease," Vascular Health and Risk Management 5, no. 1 (2009): 89–95.
8. AllSands, "What Is Obesity?" http://www.allsands.com/health/diseases/whatisobesity_wgg_gn.htm.
9. The Medical News, "Thin People May Be Obese on the Inside," May 14, 2007, http://www.news-medical.net/news/2007/05/14/25076.aspx.
10. The Harvard Medical School Family Health Guide, "Abdominal Fat and What to Do about It," updated February 2007, https://www.health.harvard.edu/fhg/updates/Abdominal-fat-and-what-to-do-about-it.shtml.
11. R. E. Ostlund, M. Staten, W. M. Kohrt, J. Schultz, and M. Malley, "The Ratio of Waist-to-Hip Circumference, Plasma Insulin Level, and Glucose Intolerance as Independent Predictors of the HDL2 Cholesterol Level in Older Adults," The New England Journal of Medicine 322, no. 4 (1990): 229–34.
12. See note 10 above.
13. R. A. Whitmer, S. Sidney, J. Selby, S. C. Johnston, and K. Yaffe, "Midlife Cardiovascular Risk Factors and Risk of Dementia in Late Life," Neurology 64, no. 2 (2005): 277–81.
14. See note 1 above.
15. S. Yusuf, S. Hawken, et al. "Obesity and the Risk of Myocardial Infarction in 27,000 Participants from 52 Countries; A Case-Control Study," Lancet, 366 (2005): 1640–49.
16. Waist-to-Hip Ratio Calculator, http://www.rush.edu/itools/hip/hipcalc.html.

17. "Modest Gain in Visceral Fat Causes Dysfunction of Blood Vessel Lining in Lean Healthy Humans; Shedding Weight Restores Vessel Health," presented by the Mayo Clinic team at the American Heart Association's Scientific Sessions, November 2007, http://www.sciencedaily.com/releases/2007/11/071105121934.htm.

Chapter 3

1. S. J. Nicholls, P. Lundman, J. A. Harmer, B. Cutri, K. A. Griffiths, K. A. Rye, P. J. Barter, and D. S. Celermajer, "Consumption of Saturated Fat Impairs the Anti-Inflammatory Properties of High-Density Lipoproteins and Endothelial Function," Journal of the American College of Cardiology 48, no. 4 (2006): 715–20.

2. D. Kritchevsky, "History of Recommendations to the Public about Dietary Fat," The Journal of Nutrition 128, no. 2 (1998): 449S–52S.

3. US Department of Health and Human Services and US Department of Agriculture, "Nutrition and Your Health: Dietary Guidelines for Americans, 1980," http://www.health.gov/dietaryguidelines/1980thin.pdf.

4. US Department of Health and Human Services and US Department of Agriculture, "Nutrition and Your Health: Dietary Guidelines for Americans, 1995," http://www.health.gov/dietaryguidelines/dga2000/default.htm.

5. US Department of Health and Human Services and US Department of Agriculture, "Nutrition and Your Health: Dietary Guidelines for Americans, 2000," http://www.health.gov/dietaryguidelines/dga2000/document/frontcover.htm.

6. US Department of Health and Human Services and US Department of Agriculture, "Nutrition and Your Health: Dietary Guidelines for Americans, 2005," http://www.health.gov/dietaryguidelines/dga2005/document/default.htm.

7. T. Thom, N. Haase, W. Rosamond, V. J. Howard, J. Rumsfeld, T. Manolio, and Z. J. Zheng, et al., "Heart Disease and Stroke Statistics—2006 Update: A Report from the American Heart Association Statistics Committee and Stroke Statistics Subcommittee," Circulation 113 no. 6 (2006): e85-e151.

8. Centers for Disease Control and Prevention, "National Health and Nutrition Examination Survey," updated August 27, 2009, http://www.cdc.gov/nchs/nhanes.htm.

9. A. Keys, C. Aravanis, H. W. Blackburn, F. S. Van Buchem, R. Buzina, B. D. Djordjevic, and A. S. Dontas, et al., "Epidemiological Studies Related to Coronary Heart Disease: Characteristics of Men Aged 40-59 in Seven Countries," Acta Medica Scandinavica, Supplementum 460 (1996): 1–392.

10. M. D. Kontogianni, D. B. Panagiotakos, C. Chrysohoou, C. Pitsavos, A. Zampelas, and C. Stefanadis, "The Impact of Olive Oil Consumption Pattern on the Risk of Acute Coronary Syndromes: The Cardio2000 Case–Control Study," Clinical Cardiology 30, no. 3 (2007): 125–29.

11. H. M. Roche, A. Zampelas, J. M. Knapper, D. Webb, C. Brooks, K. G. Jackson, and J. W. Wright, et al., "Effect of Long-Term Olive Oil Dietary Intervention on Postprandial Triacylglycerol and Factor VII Metabolism," The American Journal of Clinical Nutrition 68, no. 3 (1998): 552–60.

12. National Institutes of Health, "How You Can Lower Your Cholesterol Level," http://www.nhlbi.nih.gov/chd/lifestyles/htm.

13. C. Romero, E. Medina, J. Vargas, M. Brenes, and A. De Castro, "In Vitro Activity of Olive Oil Polyphenols against Helicobacter pylori," Journal of Agricultural and Food Chemistry 55, no. 3 (2007): 680–6.

14. K. Miura, J. Stamler, H. Nakagawa, P. Elliot, H. Ueshima, Q. Chan, and I. J. Brown, et

al., "International Study of Macro-Micronutrients and Blood Pressure Research Group," *Hypertension* 52, no. 2 (2008): 408–14.

15. N. Z. Unlu, T. Bohn, S. K. Clinton, and S. J. Schwartz, "Carotenoid Absorption from Salad and Salsa by Humans Is Enhanced by the Addition of Avocado or Avocado Oil," *The Journal of Nutrition* 135, no. 3 (2005): 431–6.

16. D. Mozaffarian and R. Clarke, "Quantitative Effects on Cardiovascular Risk Factors and Coronary Heart Disease Risk of Replacing Partially Hydrogenated Vegetable Oils with Other Fats and Oils," *European Journal of Clinical Nutrition* 63 (2009): S22–S33.

17. W. R. Archer, B. Lamarche, A. C. St-Pierre, J. F. Mauger, O. Deriaz, N. Landry, L. Corneau, J. P. Despres, J. Bergeron, J. Couture, and N. Bergeron, "High Carbohydrate and High Monounsaturated Fatty Acid Diets Similarly Affect LDL Electrophoretic Characteristics in Men Who Are Losing Weight," *The Journal of Nutrition* 133, no. 10 (2003): 3124–9.

18. L. J. Appel, F. M. Sacks, V. J. Carey, E. Obarzanek, J. F. Swain, E. R. Miller III, and P. R. Conlin, et al., for the OmniHeart Collaborative Research Group, "Effects of Protein, Monounsaturated Fat, and Carbohydrate Intake on Blood Pressure and Serum Lipids: Results of the OmniHeart Randomized Trial," *The Journal of the American Medical Association* 294, no. 19 (2005): 2455–64.

19. P. M. Kris-Etherton, T. A. Pearson, Y. Wan, R. L. Hargrove, K. Moriarty, V. Fishell, and T. D. Etherton, "High-Monounsaturated Fatty Acid Diets Lower Both Plasma Cholesterol and Triacylglycerol Concentrations," *The American Journal of Clinical Nutrition* 70, no. 6 (1999): 1009–15.

20. R. Estruch, M. A. Martinez-Gonzalez, D. Corella, J. Salas-Salvado, V. Ruiz-Gutierrez, M. I. Covas, and M. Fiol, et al., for the PREDIMED Study Investigators, "Effects of a Mediterranean-Style Diet on Cardiovascular Risk Factors: A Randomized Trial," *Annals of Clinical Medicine* 145, no. 1 (2006): 1–11.

21. Mayo Clinic staff, MayoClinic.com, "Metabolic Syndrome: Tests and Diagnosis," updated June 23, 2009, http://www.mayoclinic.com/health/metabolic%20syndrome/DS00522/DSECTION=tests-and-diagnosis.

22. L. Berglund, M. Lefebre, H. N. Ginsberg, P. M. Kris-Etherton, P. J. Elmer, P. W. Stewart, and A. Ershow, et al., for the DELTA Investigators, "Comparison of Monounsaturated Fat with Carbohydrates as a Replacement for Saturated Fat in Subjects with a High Metabolic Risk Profile: Studies in the Fasting and Postprandial States," *American Journal of Clinical Nutrition* 86, no. 6 (2007): 611–20.

23. N. Tentolouris, C. Arapostathi, D. Perrea, D. Kyriaki, C. Revenas, and N. Katsilambros, "Differential Effects of Two Isoenergetic Meals Rich in Saturated or Monounsaturated Fat on Endothelial Function in Subjects with Type 2 Diabetes," *Diabetes Care* 31, no. 12 (2008): 2276–8.

24. J. A. Paniagua, A. Gallego de la Sacristana, I. Romero, A. Vidal-Puig, J. M. Latre, E. Sanchez, P. Perez-Martinez, J. Lopez-Miranda, and F. Perez-Jimenez, "Monounsaturated Fat-Rich Diet Prevents Central Body Fat Distribution and Decreases Postprandial Adiponectin Expression Induced by a Carbohydrate-Rich Diet in Insulin-Resistant Subjects," *Diabetes Care* 30, no. 7 (2007): 1717–23.

25. B. Gumbiner, C. C. Low, and P. D. Reaven, "Effects of a Monounsaturated Fatty Acid–Enriched Hypocaloric Diet on Cardiovascular Risk Factors in Obese Patients with Type 2 Diabetes," *Diabetes Care* 21, no. 1 (1998): 9–15.

26. J. Salas-Salvado, A. Garcia-Arellano, F. Estruch, F. Marquez-Sandoval, D. Corella, M. Fiol, and E. Gomez-Gracia, et al., for the PREDIMED Investigators, "Components of the Mediterranean-Type Food Pattern and Serum Inflammatory Markers among Patients at High Risk for Cardiovascular Disease," *European Journal of Clinical Nutrition* 62 (2008): 651–9.

27. K. Esposito, R. Marfella, M. Ciotola, C. Di Palo, F. Giugliano, G. Fiugliano, M. D'Armiento, F. D'Andrea, and D. Giugliano, "Effect of a Mediterranean-Style Diet on Endothelial Dysfunction and Markers of Vascular Inflammation in the Metabolic Syndrome: A Randomized Trial," The Journal of the American Medical Association 292, no. 12 (2004): 1440–6.

28. V. Solfrizzi, F. Panza, F. Torres, F. Mastroianni, A. Del Parigi, A. Venezia, and A. Capurso, "High Monounsaturated Fatty Acids Intake Protects against Age-Related Cognitive Decline," Neurology 52, no. 8 (1999): 1563–9.

29. F. Panza, V. Solfrizzi, A. M. Colacicco, A. D'Introno, C. Capurso, F. Torres, A. Del Parigi, S. Capurso, and A. Capurso, "Mediterranean Diet and Cognitive Decline," Public Health Nutrition 7, no. 7 (2004): 959–63.

30. A. E. Norrish, R. T. Jackson, S. J. Sharpe, and C. M. Skeaff, "Men Who Consume Vegetable Oils Rich in Monosaturated Fat: Their Dietary Patterns and Risk of Prostate Cancer (New Zealand)," Cancer Causes Control 11, no. 7 (2000): 609-15.

31. D. J. Kim, R. P. Gallagher, T. G. Hislop, E. J. Holowaty, G. R. Howe, M. Jain, J. R. McLaughlin, C. Z. Teh, and T. E. Rohan, "Premorbid Diet in Relation to Survival from Prostate Cancer (Canada)," Cancer Causes Control 11, no. 1 (2000): 65-77.

32. V. Solfrizzi, A. D'Introno, A. M. Colacicco, C. Capurso, R. Palasciano, S. Capurso, F. Torres, A. Capurso, and F. Panza, "Unsaturated Fatty Acids Intake and All-Causes Mortality: A 8.5-Year Follow-Up of the Italian Longitudinal Study on Aging," Experimental Gerontology 40, no. 4 (2005): 335–43.

33. J. L. Kuk, P. T. Katzmarzyk, M. Z. Nichaman, T. S. Church, S. N. Blair, and R. Ross, "Visceral Fat Is an Independent Predictor of All-Cause Mortality in Men," Obesity 14, no. 2 (2006): 336–41.

34. J. A. Paniagua, A. Gallego de la Sacristana, I. Romero, A. Vidal-Puig, J. M. Latre, E. Sanchez, P. Perez-Martinez, J. Lopez-Miranda, and F. Perez-Jimenez, "Monounsaturated Fat-Rich Diet Prevents Central Body Fat Distribution and Decreases Postprandial Adiponectin Expression Induced by a Carbohydrate-Rich Diet in Insulin-Resistant Subjects," Diabetes Care 3, no. 7 (2007): 1717–23.

35. L. S. Piers, K. Z. Walker, R. M. Stoney, M. J. Soares, and K. O'Dea, "The Influence of the Type of Dietary Fat on Postprandial Fat Oxidation Rates: Monounsaturated (Olive Oil) vs. Saturated Fat (Cream)," International Journal of Obesity 26, no. 6 (2002): 814–21.

Chapter 4

1. Doreen Virtue, Constant Craving A-Z (Carlsbad, CA: Hay House, 1999).

2. http://www.foodandmood.org/Pages/sh-survey.html

3. J. P. Block, Y. He, A. M. Zaslavsky, L. Ding, and J. Z. Ayanian, "Psychosocial Stress and Change in Weight among US Adults," American Journal of Epidemiology 170 (2009):181–92.

4. M. Laaksonen, S. Sarlio-Lähteenkorva, P. Leino-Arjas, P. Martikainen, and E. Lahelma, "Body Weight and Health Status: Importance of Socioeconomic Position and Working Conditions," Obesity Research, 13 (2005): 2169–77.

5. D. L. Sherrill, K. Kotchou, S. F. Quan, "Association of Physical Activity and Human Sleep Disorders," Archives of Internal Medicine, 158, no. 17 (September 28, 1998): 1894–98, http://archinte.ama-assn.org/cgi/reprint/158/17/1894.

6. Ann Hettinger, "Rest Assured," Prevention 59, no. 12 (December 2007).

7. See note 6 above.

8. B. A. Edimansyah, B. N. Rusli, and L. Naing, "Effects of Short Duration Stress Management Training on Self-Perceived Depression, Anxiety and Stress in Male

Automotive Assembly Workers: A Quasi-Experimental Study," *Journal of Occupational Medicine and Toxicology* 1, no. 3 (2008): 28.

9. Mayo Clinic staff, MayoClinic.com, "Belly Fat in Men: Why Weight Loss Matters," updated June 23, 2009, http://www.mayoclinic.com/health/belly-fat/MC00054.

Chapter 5

1. J. F. Hollis, C. M. Gullion, V. J. Stevens, P. J. Brantley, L. J. Appel, J. D. Ard, C. M. Champagne, et al., for the Weight Loss Maintenance Trial Research Group, "Weight Loss During the Intensive Intervention Phase of the Weight-Loss Maintenance Trial," American Journal of Preventive Medicine 35, no. 2 (2008): 118–26.

2. D. L. Helsel, J. M. Jakicic, and A. D. Otto, "Comparison of Techniques for Self-Monitoring Eating and Exercise Behaviors on Weight Loss in a Correspondence-Based Intervention," Journal of the American Dietetic Association 107, no. 10 (2007): 1807–10.

Chapter 9

1. Simon J. Marshall et al. Translating Physical Activity Recommendations Into A Pedometer-Based Step Goal: 3000 Steps In 30 Minutes. American Journal of Preventive Medicine, Volume 36, Issue 5, May 2009.

2. A Comparison Of Linear And Daily Undulating Periodized Programs With Equated Volume And Intensity For Strength, Journal Of Strength And Conditioning Research/National Strength & Conditioning Association 2002 May;16(2):250-5, http://www.ncbi.nlm.nih.gov/pubmed/11991778

3. Glass SC, Stanton DR. (2004). Self-Selected Resistance Training Intensity In Novice Weightlifters. Journal of Strength and Conditioning Research, 18(2): 324 – 327.

4. Listening To Music While Working Out Helps People With Severe Lung Disease Improve Their Fitness Levels. http://researchnews.osu.edu/archive/pdmusic.htm

5. Television Viewing And Pedometer-Determined Physical Activity Among Multiethnic Low Income Housing Residents, American Journal of Public Health, 2006 Sep;96(9):1681-5. Epub 2006 Jul 27. http://www.ncbi.nlm.nih.gov/pubmed/16873736

6. Metabolic Cost Of Free Weight Circuit Weight Training. The Journal of Sports Medicine And Physical Fitness, 2000 Jun;40(2):118-25. http://www.ncbi.nlm.nih.gov/pubmed/11034431

7. ACE Study Finds Fitness Benefits of Wearing Casual Clothing to WorkÐCasual And Comfortable Clothing Workdays Promote Increased Physical Activity, http://www.acefitness.org/media/media_display.aspx?itemid=190

8. Physical Activity In The Treatment Of Obesity (Change), http://www.acsm.org/AM/Template.cfm?Section=Home_Page&template=/CM/ContentDisplay.cfm&ContentID=4173, http://clinicaltrials.gov/ct2/show/NCT00615238

9. Crum, Alia J., and Ellen J. Langer. 2007. Mind-Set Matters: Exercise And The Placebo Effect, Psychological Science 18, no. 2: 165-171. http://dash.harvard.edu/handle/1/3196007

Chapter 10

1. Willard Bishop, "Making Healthy Eating Easier," *Shopping for Health* 2006 survey by *Prevention* magazine (2006).

index

Boldface page references indicate photographs.
Underscored references indicate boxed text and tables.

B

Bacon. See also Canadian bacon
    BLT, 122
    Spicy Linguine with Bacon and White
        Clam Sauce, 165
Bagels
    Bagel Breakfast Sandwich, 121
Balsamic vinegar
    Almond-Crusted Chicken Breasts
        with Balsamic Drizzle, 175
    Balsamic Portobello and Vegetable
        Mixed Grill, 189
Bananas
    Banana Chocolate Smoothie, 132
    Banana Split Oatmeal, 120
    Peanut Butter–Banana Smoothie, 132
    Strawberry-Banana and Pecan
        Sundaes, 196
Barbecue sauce
    Grilled Chicken Breasts with Peanut
        Barbecue Sauce, 179
Basil. See also Pesto
    Dijon Basil Chicken, 128
    Pan-Seared Salmon Fillet with
        Tomato, Basil, and Kalamata Olives,
        172
Beans
    Black and Red Bean Chili with Wagon
        Wheels, 167
    Mexican Bean and Avocado Salsa
        with Baked Tortilla Chips, 191
    Morning Mex Quesadilla, 122
    Refried Bean Wrap, 123
Beef
    Beef and Gruyère Hoagie, 123
    Cashew Beef with Broccoli and Snow
        Peas, 169
    Flank Steak Chopped Steakhouse
        Salad, 161
    Fontina Beef Pita, 124
    Grilled Filet Mignon with Grilled
        Onion and Avocado, 183
    Grilled Flank Steak with Olive Oil Mojo
        Sauce, 182
    Penne Bolognese, 164
    Pesto-Parmesan-Topped Burgers
        on Portuguese Rolls, 181
    Romaine Roast Beef Wraps with
        Horseradish Cream, 154
    Shredded "Beef" Burrito, 126
    Tex-Mex Soup, 126
Beer, xiii, 103
Beer belly, xiii, 14, 44, 60
Bell, Jimmy, 16
Belly fat
    causes of, xiii, 214, 248
    health risks from, xiv, 2, 13–14, 41
    in men, xiii, 1–2, 41
    MUFAs and, xiii–xiv, 3, 25, 41–42, 253
    types of, 2–3 (see also Subcutaneous
        fat; Visceral fat)
Berries. See also specific berries
Beverages. See also Fire Water; specific
    beverages
    calories in, 136
    during Four-Day Flat Abs Kickstart,
        79
    types to avoid, 76–77, 103
Bioelectrical impedance analysis (BIA), for
    measuring visceral fat, 20
Bloating
    causes of, 73, 77, 80
    Four-Day Flat Abs Kickstart reducing,
        73–75
    as health problem, 80
Blondies
    Macadamia Nut Blondies, 193
Blood lipids. See Cholesterol; Triglycerides
Blood pressure reduction. See also High
    blood pressure
    from Flat Belly Diet, 4
    MUFAs for, 35, 36
Blueberries
    Almond, Blueberry, and Brown Sugar
        Oatmeal, 146
BMI. See Body mass index
Body fat
    calories for gaining, 74
    excess, dangers of, 12, 18
    functions of, 11, 18
    hormones and, 15

V

Vegetables. See also specific vegetables
  Balsamic Portobello and Vegetable
    Mixed Grill, 189
  Breakfast Veggie Sandwich, 120
  Ginger Tahini Dip with Crudite, 130
  Lunch Crudites, 124
  PB Vegged Out, 130
Visceral fat, 2–3, 4, 6
  health risks from, 16–18, 21, 41
  measuring, 18–21

W

Waffles
  Waffle Sandwich, 121
  Waffle Sundae, 131
Waist measurement
  health problems linked to, 13–14, 19
  unhealthy, 18
Waist-to-hip ratio, 18–19
Walking
  after-meal, in Four-Day Flat Abs
    Kickstart, 77
  benefits of, 203, 242
  Calorie Torch Walk, 203, 204, 206,
    207, 208–11, 238–39
  Fat Blast Walk, 203, 204, 205–6, 207,
    208–11, 238–39
  for improving sleep, 56
  intensity of, 205–7, 207
  monthly plan for, 208–11
  reducing hamstring soreness from,
    206
  shoes for, 212, 213
  socks for, 212
  technique for, 212–13
  on treadmill vs. outdoors, 240
Walnut oil, health benefits of, 35
Walnuts. See also Nuts
  health benefits of, 35
Wasabi
  Lemon-Herb-Marinated Tuna Burger
    with Wasabi Aioli, 186

Water. See also Fire Water
  during exercise, 240
  plain, as alternative to Fire Water,
    79, 103
  weight fluctuations from, 74
Water retention, 74, 75, 102
Web site
  calorie information on, 119
  Flat Belly Diet for Men, 102
Weight belts, 240–41
Weight gain
  from stress, 50, 51
  from water vs. calories, 74
  work-related, 51, 55
Weight loss
  from Flat Belly Diet, xiv, xv, 4, 5
  from Four-Day Flat Abs Kickstart, 5,
    69–70, 74–75
  slowed by muscle loss, 43
Weight-loss challenges
  dealing with, 249–50
  guys' night out, 60–61, 249
  lack of family support, 63–64
  sedentary work and play, 61
  sporting events and other activities,
    61–62, 249
  stress, 50–59
  travel, 62–63, 249
Weight-loss plateaus, 250
Work
  sedentary, as weight-loss challenge, 61
  traveling for, 62–63
  weight gain from, 51, 55
Wraps. See Sandwiches

X

Xylitol, avoiding, 76

Y

Yogurt
  Nutty Breakfast Crunch, 120
  Yogurt Crunch Delight, 131

The Ultimate
Plan *to* Blast Belly Fat!

Introducing the EASIEST, BUDGET-MAXIMIZING Eating Plan Yet!

Flat Belly Diet!
Pocket Guide

LOSE UP TO 15 LBS IN 32 DAYS!

- BEST FOOD CH... ...GO
- SHOPPING LIST... ...ERS!
- MEAL M...

LIZ VACCARIE...
Coauthor ...

FREE 21-DAY PREVIEW!

The ***Flat Belly Diet! Pocket Guide*** is the must-have guide to making healthy food choices in the store, at a restaurant, and more!

This handy and user-friendly book provides *at-a-glance information*, such as:

- Best Food Choices on the Go
- Complete 28-Day Meal Plan
- Calorie Counter and Lists of Serving Sizes
- Meal Maker at a Glance
- ... and more!

Take it with you wherever you go!

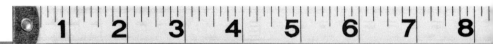

The hottest diet in America!

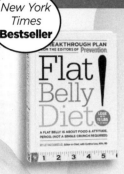

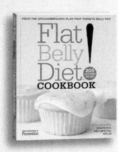

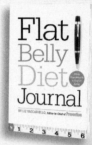

Flat Belly Diet! gives you all the tips and moves you need to eliminate belly bulge—no crunches required! A simple plan with easy-to-follow instructions, quick-fix meal plans, and delicious recipes.

Flat Belly Diet! Cookbook is for the food-lover in you, with 200 all-new seriously tasty recipes and a guide to making your own *Flat Belly Diet!*–friendly meals.

Flat Belly Diet! Journal is yo essential tool to track what eat and strengthen your da commitment to lifelong hea and vitality.

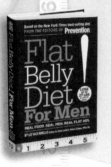

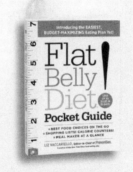

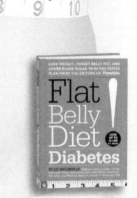

Flat Belly Diet! for Men Adapted for men's needs and appetites. In addition to MUFAs, the diet incorporates protein to boost testosterone and fiber to keep hungry men satisfied. Calorie levels are also adjusted that men can lose weight without feeling hungry.

Flat Belly Diet! Pocket Guide is a handy and user-friendly book that enables you to make healthy food choices at restaurants and wherever you go in the store.

Flat Belly Diet! Diabetes Yo can lose your belly fat, eras stubborn pounds and can p yourself on the road to bett blood sugar and less risk fo diabetes. With super-satisfy treats in the mix of healthy foods you'll eat at every me

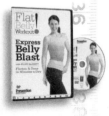

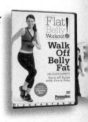

The Flat Belly Workout! Express Belly Blast DVD is a combination cardio, toning, and yoga program that will help you burn fat, boost metabolism, and beat stress— the hidden cause of belly flab.

The Flat Belly Workout! Walk Off Belly Fat DVD is an easy-to-follow 25-minute indoor workout that combines simple walking moves with torso-toning exercises.